Colds & Coughs

Jim Glenn

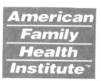

American Family Health Institute™

Medical Board

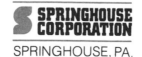

SPRINGHOUSE CORPORATION

SPRINGHOUSE, PA.

The charter of the American Family Health Institute is to research and produce high-quality publications that enhance the health of individuals and their families. Essential to health are physical, emotional, and social well-being, not just the absence of illness or infirmity. The Institute's Medical Board has produced the *Health and Fitness* books to share up-to-date and authoritative information that can give readers greater personal control over their health maintenance.

Library of Congress Cataloging-in-Publication Data
Glenn, Jim.

    Colds & coughs.

    (Health & fitness)
    Includes index.
    1. Cold (Disease)—Popular works.   2.
Cough.   I. Dudrick, Stanley J.   II.
American Family Health Institute. Medical
Board.   III. Title.   IV. Title: Colds and
coughs.   V. Series: Health and fitness
series. [DNLM: 1. Common Cold—popular
works. 2. Cough—popular works. WC 510
G558c]
RF361.G57   1986   616.2'05   86-14340
ISBN 0-87434-071-3

The procedures and explanations given in this publication are based on research and consultation with medical and nursing authorities. To the best of our knowledge, these procedures and explanations reflect currently accepted medical practice; nevertheless, they can't be considered absolute and universal recommendations. For individual application, treatment suggestions must be considered in light of the individual's health, subject to a doctor's specific recommendations. The authors and the publisher disclaim responsibility for any adverse effects resulting directly or indirectly from the suggested procedures, from any undetected errors, or from the reader's misunderstanding of the text.

Contents

Colds & Coughs

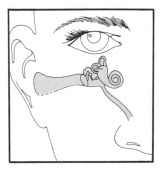

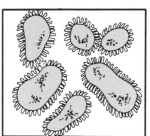

1

Medical Knowledge about Colds

Your cold, defined
Here's a concise medical description of a cold: "An acute, usually afebrile, catarrhal respiratory tract infection, with major involvement in any or all airways, including the nose, paranasal passages, throat, larynx, and often the trachea and bronchi." What do these phrases mean? Three major things: Colds bring little or no fever (afebrile), cause increased mucus flow (catarrhal), and may affect tissues from your nose to your lungs and anywhere in between. Notice that a specific infectious agent isn't mentioned. A cold's symptoms are distinctive but its causes aren't, because the cause can be any one of several hundred viral strains.

For centuries, people have suffered from the common cold, unable to point to its cause. Today, specialists can describe with some precision what causes colds. They've made discoveries, too, about how colds spread from person to person, who are the likeliest targets, how colds can lead to more serious illness. But specialists still can't tell you how to get rid of a cold once you've caught it.

What is a cold?

The common cold is the most common illness suffered by humans. If you don't have a cold right now, you're almost sure to get one within the next 12 months. Because we all have colds occasionally, we know what we mean when we talk about this illness. If it weren't for our common experience with colds, however, defining colds would be next to impossible.

Colds are viral infections, but they're caused by several hundred distinct viruses belonging to several different viral families. To further complicate things, your short bout with flu viruses or other viruses can produce symptoms identical to those of more common cold viruses. Only when your symptoms progress in particular ways can anyone know whether you have a cold or the flu.

Cold symptoms vary enormously. The usual symptoms include sneezing, sinus congestion, runny nose, sore throat, cough, low fever, and headache. If you experience any combination of these symptoms, you'll probably believe you've caught a cold. Of course, your conclusion could be incorrect: the same symptoms could signal the beginnings of another illness— whooping cough, influenza, strep throat, or even an allergy. Sooner or later, if your symptoms worsen, if they don't disappear when you think they should, or if uncoldlike symptoms show up, you'll stop believing you have a cold and start considering other diseases.

Cold symptoms result from your body's defense against infection. The inflammation that causes most of a cold's symptoms is part of that defense process. Doctors think of a cold as a syndrome—a group of symptoms that reach a certain severity and last a certain time. To say that you have a cold is, in a

Other names for a cold
Two terms describing colds go back hundreds of years. Now seen mostly in medical books, catarrh and coryza were once common ways of naming a runny nose. Both terms derive from Greek roots meaning essentially the same thing, "increased flow."

Cold symptoms: What and where

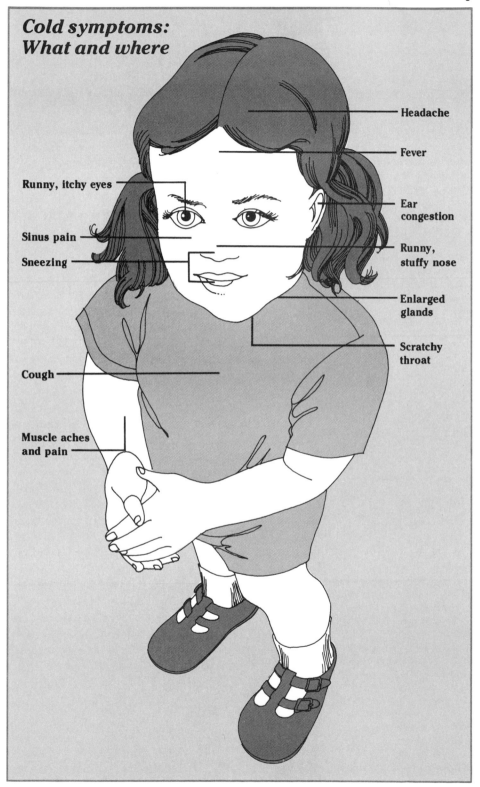

Headache

Fever

Ear congestion

Runny, stuffy nose

Enlarged glands

Scratchy throat

Runny, itchy eyes

Sinus pain

Sneezing

Cough

Muscle aches and pain

Virus—a poison

Hardly flattering, the term virus *is taken from Latin meaning "a slimy liquid or poison." Viruses aren't slimy liquids, of course, but received their name at the turn of the century: medical researchers found that viruses could transmit diseases in filtered fluids that were free of bacteria, protozoa, funguses, and other known disease agents. What was left was invisible under the best microscopes of the time. Invisible or not, these laboratory fluids did cause disease, so scientists simply named the still-unidentified culprits a poison, a virus.*

The bacteria balance

We live in a generally stable balance with bacteria both inside and outside the body. We are constantly exposed to quite harmful bacteria (most are permanent residents of our skin), yet we aren't very often infected. The arrangement is a complex one; no one has yet fully explained how a healthy balance is struck between us and bacteria, or how the balance breaks.

special sense, to say that your immune system is in action. If your symptoms go away soon enough, you won't need more expert opinions about your infection. So you'll finally and definitely label the recent skirmish between your body and an unknown, unpleasant invader a cold.

Bacteria

For a clearer understanding of cold infections, we should take a closer look at the cause, viruses. We'll begin by distinguishing viruses from another common infection cause, bacteria.

Bacteria are a life form. Single-celled organisms, they feed, breathe, reproduce, expel wastes, and die, as do all life forms. Judged by their genetic makeup, bacteria are closely related to plants. They're present in all living things. Many bacteria are useful, even essential, to other, larger life forms, including us— like so many life forms, from insects to mammals, we need bacteria for digestion. We also use bacteria in other ways: for preparing cheese, manufacturing synthetic materials and drugs, feeding on waste oil sludge.

Bacteria harmful to our health are, thankfully, relatively few when compared to the thousands of bacterial species around us. That still leaves scores of bacteria potentially dangerous to humans. Once, these bacteria caused epidemics, prolonged suffering, and death. Since the development of antibiotics, we hold the upper hand in treating bacterial infection— we're not always successful, but we no longer live in fear of raging bacterial disease. The combination of proper hygiene and antibiotics has probably done more than any other medical measure to lengthen our lives.

Bacteria don't cause colds, but they can cause symptoms you may confuse with a cold. If you have a bacterial infection with cough, sore throat, or other coldlike symptoms, you should see a doctor. Be sure to read Chapter 5 to help you determine whether your symptoms might identify a bacterial disease.

Viruses

Viruses may well be the simplest, barest biochemicals that can, in the right environment, copy themselves exactly. A typical virus, only a few ten-billionths of an inch long (much smaller than bacteria), consists of two chief parts: a geometrically regular and com-

Where you may pick up a virus at work

You'll have plenty of opportunities to encounter viral infection in your office or workplace. You may have little choice in your schedule and mode of travel. Frequent hand washing is your most effective defense. A clean, well-ventilated office environment also contributes to your continuing good health. Here are some danger points:

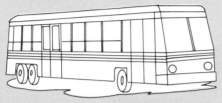

Public transportation—Buses, subways, and trains are confined, stuffy environments where you will be exposed to illness carried by fellow passengers.

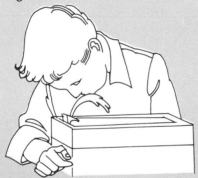

Water fountains and bathroom facilities—Faucet handles and fountain knobs are chief offenders.

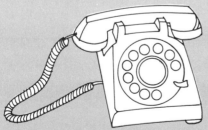

Telephones—These instruments can carry an amazing contaminant load. They are constantly handled and virtually drenched in moisture and contaminant-laden breath. Disinfectant sprays for telephones may help.

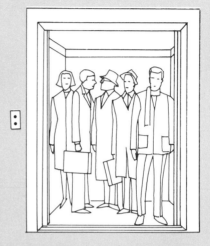

Elevators—You travel face to face in these poorly ventilated, crowded places. Better conditions for transmitting a virus can scarcely be imagined.

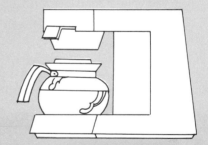

Office coffee machines—Any office appliance used by everyone should be treated with suspicion. Covered cup dispensers are a must; sugar and cream containers must be protected, too. Your defenses against office contagion are limited.

pact protein coat and an interior packed with RNA or DNA. All life forms contain the genetic materials RNA and DNA. But life forms also have many other essential components to clean, rebuild, and power their cells. Viruses don't breathe, produce energy or wastes, or feed in any conventional sense. They reproduce in such a streamlined, primitive way that we call the process *replication*.

Harmful bacteria affect us in several different ways: through powerful toxins (poisons) they release, through accumulation of bacterial waste products, or through direct cell invasion. Viral damage is always the same because viruses must enter and destroy cells in order to replicate themselves.

A virus's protective outer shell is a simple affair as biological structures go. No frills: it keeps viral genetic material in and most damaging substances out. Small sections of the coat are chemically coded to attach themselves to one kind of living cell, usually within only one kind of host. For example, some viruses recognize only certain blood cells in mice, others a particular plant's leaf tissue. Even bacteria can be viral targets. The many viruses that cause the common cold happen to need cells like those in our throats.

Once a virus has found its target, it forces its way through the cell wall. Inside the cell, the virus's protective coat dissolves, spilling the virus's neatly packed inner parts—its genetic material—into the host cell. The virus ransacks the cell's contents for raw materials to manufacture new viruses. Generally, a few hours pass before new viruses begin to "bud" outward through the infected cell's wall. The ruptured, depleted cell dies, releasing hundreds of new viruses to infect hundreds more cells.

If your body had no defenses against such an invasion, cell destruction would continue until the virus could find no more suitable cells. Fortunately, your body has excellent defenses, and a viral infection rarely continues unchecked.

Viral families linked to colds

Eight different viral families are estimated to cause between 60% and 70% of all colds. That 30% to 40% of colds haven't been pinned down to known viruses isn't surprising: even with modern biochemical techniques and powerful electron microscopes, detecting

The viral world
About 40 virus groups are disease causers in man. Easily the most common are the respiratory viruses—those that cause colds, flu, mumps, and infectious mononucleosis. Luckily for us, very few viruses get around as easily as cold viruses. That's why you don't have to worry about catching, say, Rift Valley fever or Kyasanur Forest disease at the office. Like most viruses, these require a more complex transmission method than mere sneezing.

Comparing bacteria and viruses

Description	Traits	Harmful effects	Treatment
Bacteria			
single-celled life form	• reproduce (by dividing) • breathe • feed and produce energy • often mobile	• produce toxins and wastes • kill cells • attack a broad range of cell types	• antibiotics usually effective
Viruses			
subcellular; usually not considered "alive"	• self-copying (sometimes viruses divide but usually assemble copies within infected cells) • don't breathe • don't feed • don't produce energy • no means of locomotion	• invade cells, but are usually very specialized, seeking a narrow range of suitable cell types	• antibiotics have no effect • new antiviral drugs work against a limited number • vaccines, if available, still most powerful weapon

Viral multitudes

A single virus, using the materials available in a single infected cell, may produce thousands of copies of itself. Fortunately, few viruses can accomplish this production-line feat in fewer than 4 to 6 hours—giving your immune system time to act. Viral replication kills healthy cells. Fortunately, though, viruses aren't efficient in their self-copying process: a large percentage of the viral copies are defective and don't pose any threat to body cells.

the tiniest viruses challenges our technology. In addition, some colds are minor bouts with more serious infection—viruses caught in the respiratory tract before they can reach other, preferred body tissues.

The eight chief cold virus groups, though very different from one another, find the respiratory tract a suitable environment for copying themselves. Some of these viruses can find other targets in the body. More specialized viruses, however, are usually harmless anywhere beyond your nose and throat. On rare occasions, these viruses can cause severe, atypical illness—anything from paralysis to brain infection. No one knows why this happens.

—Rhinovirus, the most common cold virus, appears in over a hundred known varieties. Scientists suspect a full list would run into hundreds more. Rhinovirus

(continued on page 12)

"Seeing" a virus

Viruses are so small you can't see one under an ordinary microscope. A virus just doesn't exist as far as ordinary light is concerned; anything of viral size won't reflect or interfere with visible light in any way that leads to a useful picture.

How do scientists "see" viruses? They use electron beams in electron microscopes that magnify viruses by powers of several hundred thousand. These illustrations, adapted from microscopic photos, show viruses magnified about 200,000 times.

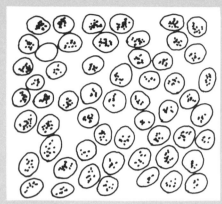

Rhinovirus

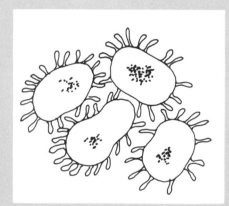

Coronavirus

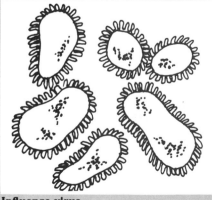

Influenza virus

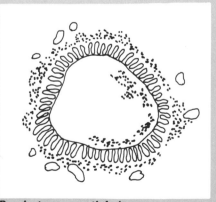

Respiratory syncytial virus

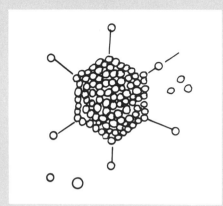

Adenovirus

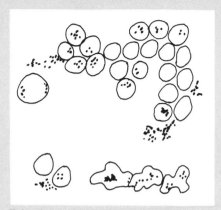

Echovirus

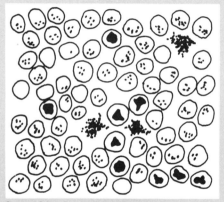

Coxsackie virus

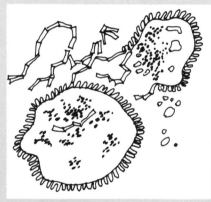

Parainfluenza virus

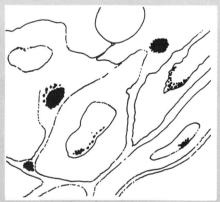

Herpes simplex virus

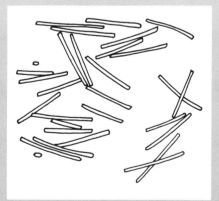

Tobacco mosaic virus

rarely causes anything more than an uncomplicated cold.

Along with echovirus and Coxsackie virus, rhinovirus belongs to the tiniest kinds of virus, only 2 or 3 billionths of an inch across. Of course, even comparative giants among the cold viruses, such as parainfluenza, are still unimaginably small—no more than 12 or 14 billionths of an inch at most.

—Coronavirus is runner-up to rhinovirus in giving us colds. This virus flourishes at the peak of the cold season, during winter months. Coronavirus, among the most recently discovered cold viruses, is named for the crownlike rays, or spikes, projecting in a regular array from its spherical shell. (*Corona* means

What happens when a virus attacks

A virus that attacks a cell sheds its protective coat and takes control of the cell. The cell then produces new viruses that attack other cells. At the same time, though, the controlled cell also produces interferon, a substance that helps other cells produce antiviral proteins. These proteins can block the spreading virus' commands.

Unfortunately, interferon has a limited effect and slows the viral spread for only the first few days of an infection.

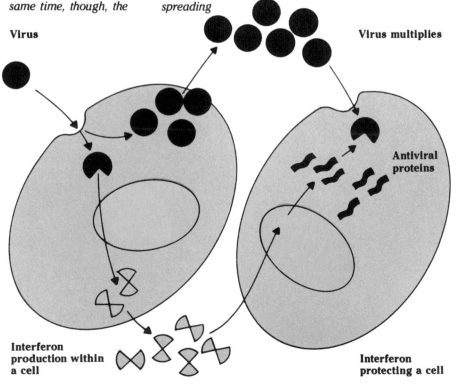

Virus

Virus multiplies

Antiviral proteins

Interferon production within a cell

Interferon protecting a cell

"crown" in Latin.)

—Adenovirus affects chiefly children, but several of its 33 strains cause adult illnesses. Adenovirus colds can be severe, with fever and eye infection, and this virus is active all year.

Curiously, adenovirus often brings with it another, smaller virus, called AAV (adeno-associated virus), that seems to depend on adenovirus to help it copy itself.

—Echovirus belongs to the summer and fall. Its 28 strains usually infect infants and children, producing symptoms other than colds, such as fever and diarrhea. Still, echovirus shows up regularly in colds.

—Coxsackie virus, named after a New York town where it was first identified, resembles echovirus. Coxsackie's 30 known strains may also produce intestinal symptoms, mostly in the very young, and colds with fever.

—Respiratory syncytial virus (RSV) causes generally mild colds in adults but occasionally brings more flulike symptoms. Very young children experience more serious illness, often deep in the respiratory tract. RSV prefers late fall and winter, but it has only one strain.

—Influenza (flu) virus has three very different strains: A, B, and C. All cause colds as well as flu, but type A is responsible for the most serious flu outbreaks. Influenza virus, like parainfluenza, may appear as croup in children. Both viruses bring a risk of serious complication, pneumonia.

—Parainfluenza virus doesn't spread well except among children—most adults have immunity. One or another of its four strains is active year-round.

2

How Your Body Fights Infection

Why doesn't your immune system attack you?
All your body's cells are "tagged" with a special protein that is unique to you. The protein's blueprint is carried in your genes. When components of your immune system encounter your particular protein, they recognize the cell and don't attack. When someone else's protein shows up in your body, after a skin graft or an organ transplant, your immune system may well attack and "reject" the new part.

Defective T cells may attack the body they're meant to protect, causing an autoimmune disease. The long list of autoimmune disorders includes some types of arthritis, anemia, multiple sclerosis, thyroid disease, acquired immunodeficiency syndrome, and others.

Your body tries to keep you infection-free by cleaning the air you breathe. Your respiratory tract performs this task by continuously sweeping away dirt and microbes with mucus produced along the whole length of your air passages. Besides this effective mucous protection, you have powerful biochemical defenses at work within the tissues themselves. Active anti-infection agents circulate continually in your bloodstream and lymph vessels. We refer to them collectively as the immune system.

Your immune system

To protect you from infection, your immune system responds to bacterial and viral invaders. At the same time, it must recognize—and not disturb—the helpful bacteria that live naturally inside you, such as those that live in the intestines and aid digestion. A healthy immune system carries out three vital functions:
—alerting uninfected areas of an invasion
—identifying potentially harmful organisms
—organizing an effective defense, providing both fast, general measures and slower, specific responses.

If you're invaded by a cold virus and your immune system carries out all three of its functions well, you can look forward to a speedy recovery, though not necessarily a painless one. The measures your immune system takes to fight infection cause your cold's symptoms.

The alert

A bacterial or viral invader destroys healthy body cells. But even while they're being destroyed, the first infected cells alert the rest of your body to the invader's presence. The attacked cells release a substance called interferon. This substance circulates to nearby unaffected cells and stimulates them to produce proteins that defend them from the virus. Your body's immune system, alerted to the virus' presence, begins a defense. At this stage, you're still blissfully unaware of what's taking place.

Other proteins spill from the infected cells and attract attention from specialized immune cells called mast cells; mast cells store substances called mediators. These mediators cause inflammation by bringing

Endless antibodies

The antibody molecule is amazingly versatile. These Y-shaped proteins can produce as many as a billion distinct variations, in theory. With this kind of flexibility, your immune system should find an effective weapon against any invader—given a little time. In fact, the few diseases that defy the immune system usually have developed complex strategies to disguise themselves. Such sophisticated diseases (like some forms of malaria or filariasis) might change their outer coats frequently or clothe themselves in their host's own proteins, thus misleading the immune system.

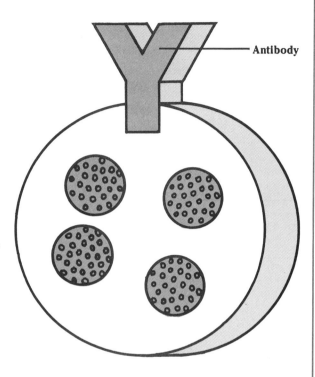

Antibody

Mast cell

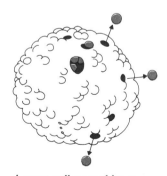

A mast cell resembles a spherical seedpod—only the mast cell releases tiny histamine particles that initiate your body's inflammatory response to a foreign presence in the body.

fluids and blood to the infected area and increasing mucus production. At this stage, you may know—from your swelling nasal passages—that something is amiss.

Inflammation isn't directed at any particular invader. It works well as a first defense, sweeping away microorganisms in mucus and bringing more specialized blood agents to the scene. At this stage, your fever may begin.

Of the body's various inflammatory responses, fever's function is least understood. Apparently, parts of the immune defense work better at higher temperature. Interferon and some white blood cells, particularly, are more active at fever temperatures. On the other hand, a fever means that your heart beats faster and works a little harder. Extreme fevers (over 104° F.) can harm the brain and therefore must be treated as emergencies.

Fever, swelling, congestion, sneezing, and coughing

Viral geometry

Rhinovirus, like many other viruses, is a regular geometric solid—in this case a 20-sided solid, called an icosahedron. Rhinovirus's 20 faces have recently been deciphered by researchers. Each protein building block in the viral structure has now been exactly located and identified. With this knowledge, we're that much closer to discovering new ways of blocking or destroying the virus.

will have certainly alerted you to an invader's presence. Your symptoms have also alerted your body's disease specialists, the white blood cells. As they arrive in increasing numbers at the infected site, they will identify the invader and further your defense.

Identification

Your blood contains many cells with special functions. Red blood cells outnumber other cells; they carry oxygen throughout your body. White blood cells are your body's defenders. (They're called white blood cells because they're colorless under a microscope.) Small, jagged platelets, also quite numerous, help in blood clotting. Other substances, like nutrients, proteins, and enzymes, circulate continuously, being used as needed by body cells.

Of the means our bodies have created to fight disease, perhaps the strangest is the monocyte. Like other white blood cells, the monocyte comes into being inside bone marrow. After entering the blood stream and migrating for a while, it undergoes a transformation, emerging as a macrophage (Greek for "big eater"). Macrophages engulf any foreign substance they encounter in the blood, even worn-out or defective red blood cells. Viruses and bacteria, too, are in the macrophage diet. Somehow, macrophages not only digest viruses but also report on them to some other white blood cells, which act on this information.

Another kind of white blood cell, the lymphocyte, comes in two varieties, T cells and B cells. A T cell collects information from a macrophage when it comes into contact with one. The T cell orchestrates the most elaborate of our three immune stages, the defense.

Defense

The big eaters do more than communicate an invader's identity; they also destroy viruses. In fact, macrophages energetically feed at an infected site, and they reproduce quickly. But even a macrophage's appetite can't cope with a quickly self-copying virus. T cells, however, use strategies less primitive than merely eating the adversary.

T cells

T cells are created in tens of thousands of close variations to one another. Only a few T cells will recognize and act on the biochemical information carried by a macrophage that has eaten a particular kind of virus.

The lymphatic system

Disease-fighting cells are located at strategic points within your body. Together, these form the lymphatic system. The tonsils and adenoids are lymphatic structures; other major parts of the lymphatic system are lymph nodes—located, for example, in the neck, armpits, and upper thighs (groin). The thymus, in your chest, is the lymphatic system's master control gland. The spleen, appendix, Peyer's patches, and tonsils help the lymph nodes.

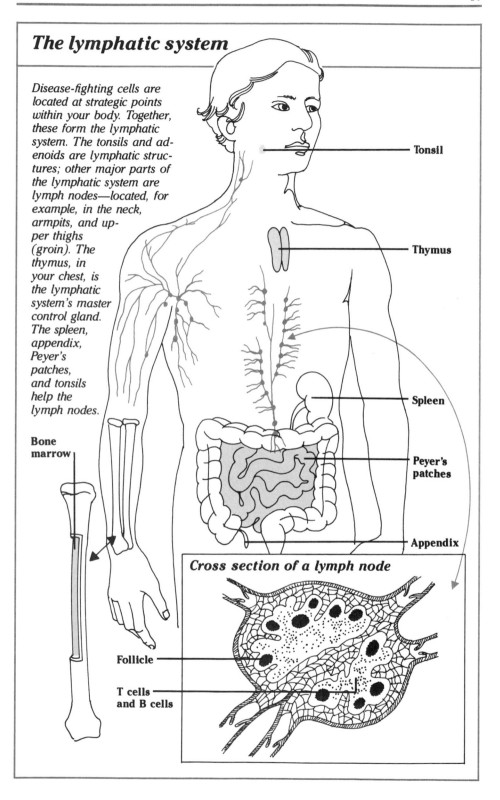

Tonsil

Thymus

Spleen

Peyer's patches

Appendix

Bone marrow

Cross section of a lymph node

Follicle

T cells and B cells

Inflammation

When your body senses disease or injury, its first response is usually inflammation, which you'll feel as swelling (or perhaps throbbing) and warmth in the affected parts. Increased fluid in the spaces between cells causes the swelling; histamine can activate swelling, as can other substances called mediators. Warmth reflects greater blood supply to diseased or damaged areas. The inflammation brings nutrients and antibodies to the trouble site and carries away damaged cells.

Those T cells that do recognize the message take action. First, they secrete a more specific and effective interferon—one that will aid as yet uninfected cells to repel the now identified virus. Other immediate T cell responses include attracting and activating other white blood cells.

Next, T cells divide quickly and repeatedly into four kinds of "daughter" T cells: killer, helper, suppressor, and memory T cells. Killer T cells destroy body cells that the virus has entered, catching the virus at a vulnerable stage.

Antibodies

Helper T cells bring information to another kind of lymphocyte, the B cells. Acting on clues supplied both by T cells and macrophages, B cells begin to produce antibodies. Antibodies are your body's most advanced weapon against viruses and other harmful

How a virus is destroyed

When a killer T cell attacks a virus-infected cell, the killer T cell releases proteins that destroy the infected cell's contents.

THE ATTACK BEGINS

Virus-infected cell

Killer T cell

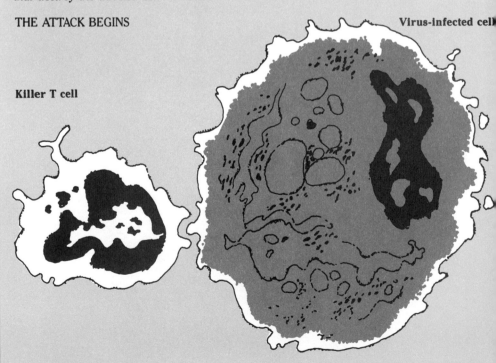

organisms. These substances are tailored to block a particular invader.

An antibody needn't be very large or complex. They're all variations on a basic design that B cells can turn out quickly and in great numbers. Antibodies simply attach themselves to a virus or bacterium, blunting the organism's ability to force entry into a healthy cell. Later, the neutralized virus will be broken up by blood substances known as complements. A complement consists of nine distinct, active proteins and nine inhibitor proteins that deactivate the first group when they finish destructive work.

Mopping up

Suppressor T cells come into action as the battle ends. As evidence of infection grows scarcer, suppressor T

(continued on page 22)

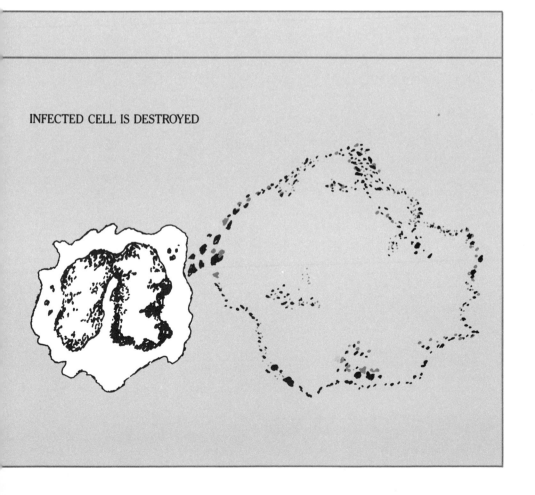

INFECTED CELL IS DESTROYED

Understanding fever

The hypothalamus regulates your body temperature. When inflammation begins (with an infected sinus, for example), your hypothalamus takes its cue from a mediator that's released by your immune response. Though not yet fully identified, this mediator is called endogenous pyrogen.

After receiving the mediator signal, the hypothalamus takes steps to raise your body's metabolism, increasing heart and breathing rates. The resulting higher body temperature stimulates components of your immune system:

macrophages and T cells become more active, reproducing more quickly.

Though you've heard that 98.6° F. is a normal temperature, in reality that's an average. Normal temperature varies with time of day and from person to person. Temperatures from 97.8° to 99.2° F. are within the normal range. You have a fever when your temperature rises above 100° F. At 102° F. (103° F. in children), you should see a doctor. As fever passes 104° F., danger to your health increases quickly.

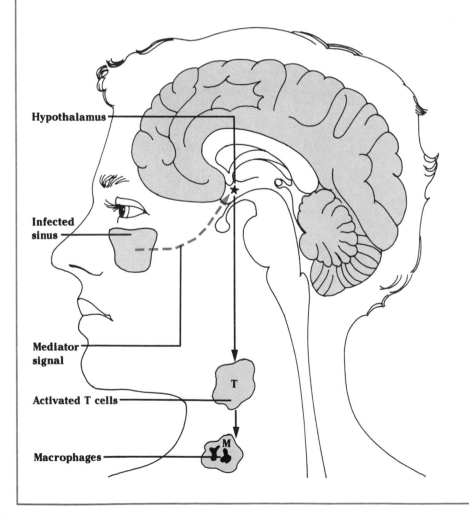

Hypothalamus

Infected sinus

Mediator signal

Activated T cells

Macrophages

How to check body temperature

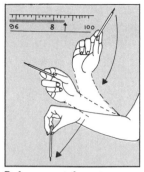

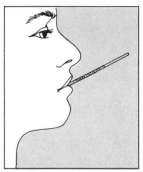

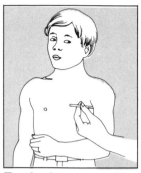

Before you take a temperature, shake the mercury down with several sharp flicks of your wrist. Then wash the thermometer in cool water.

If a sick child can hold the thermometer under his tongue and won't bite it (usually children over age 6 or 7), slip the bulb of the thermometer under his tongue. Then have him close his mouth. You can also use this method to take your own temperature.

To take the temperature of a child who can't use an oral thermometer, put the bulb in one armpit, and fold the forearm across the child's chest.

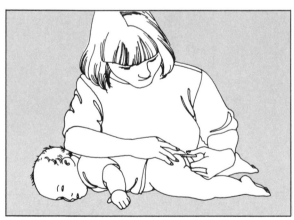

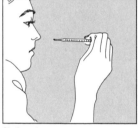

To take an infant's or toddler's temperature, place the infant or toddler on his stomach. Using your arm and elbow to control his movements, spread the *infant's buttocks open and insert the bulb of a special rectal thermometer about 1½ inches into his rectum.*

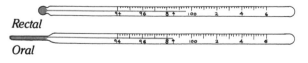

Rectal

Oral

If the thermometer was in the mouth, remove it after 3 minutes; in the armpit, after 10 minutes; in the rectum, after 3 minutes.

Hold the thermometer up to the light and turn it slowly until you see the top of the mercury column. This is the person's temperature. (For temperatures taken under the armpit, add 1° F. to the reading to equal the temperature you would have gotten with an oral thermometer. For temperatures taken in the rectum, subtract 1° F.)

Why "T" and "B"

T cells are named for the thymus, the gland in which they mature. B cells are a more complicated matter— named for an anatomical structure found only in birds, not in humans. That anatomical feature is the bursa of Fabricius, and B cells develop there. Until recently, medical scientists couldn't say for certain where B cells in humans originate. Evidence now strongly suggests their production in the fetal liver as well as in bone marrow and the intestinal lining.

cells begin to turn off the immune response, slowing the macrophages and damping the activity of B cells and other T cells.

Memory T cells remain. They will circulate in the blood for years, looking always for something they recognize—the particular invader that brought them into existence. Antibodies, too, and memory B cells (similar to memory T cells) will circulate long after your illness has disappeared. That's one reason why you're well more often than sick. Your body's assorted antibodies destroy most viruses before any symptoms can appear.

Immunity

You've probably heard that you never catch the same cold twice. Doctors believe this is pretty much true. Indeed, you may not catch that cold's nearest relative either.

Even though the viruses of a single family may number hundreds of variants, an antibody created to fight one often serves to disable a few other strains. In this way, your circulating antibodies give you a little more immunity for each disease they successfully beat off. This effect explains your generally lower incidence of colds as you grow older. Your immune system can identify more disease organisms and act against them more quickly.

Viruses can alter their biochemical appearance rapidly, presenting new faces to antibodies. Sometimes the change is enough to evade the immune system's recognition—and you'll have another cold.

3

The Classic Cold

The only thing "as easy as catching a cold" is getting advice on how to rid yourself of this illness. But you know from experience that you can't cure a cold. You can, however, do a few things to make yourself more comfortable while you wait to recover your health.

Who gets colds

While you're sneezing, aching, and dining on hot chicken soup, you'll probably ask yourself if you did something to deserve this. Why you? Are colds going around at the office? Too much stress and too little sleep lately? Or were you overdue for a cold because you hadn't had one yet this year?

A "yes" answer to any of these questions—or to all three—could have some bearing on why you got your cold. You'll never know for sure. Colds do tend to infect people near a cold sufferer; they do seem to pick on people under stress; and they do occur more or less regularly, though not predictably, throughout our lives.

No one has actually counted the number of colds Americans catch each year, but based on the average incidence of colds, we can estimate that the number is at least a half a billion each year. Most colds last from a week to 10 days, taking students out of school 2 days for each cold and workers away from their jobs an average of half a day for each cold. This makes colds a very big business—mostly the business of over-the-counter (OTC), or nonprescription, remedies and doctor visits. Though we invest about $500 million each year in cold medicines, we know we're not curing the disease, just hoping to relieve the symptoms. Unfortunately, we may fail even at obtaining relief. Long-term studies by the U.S. Food and Drug Administration (FDA) tested the effects of over 200 OTC remedies and found that most of these products can't do what their labels claim.

Besides looking at cures, scientists have viewed colds from nearly every possible angle. They've photographed viruses, cataloged symptoms, inoculated volunteers both with cold viruses and vaccines, and compiled statistics about who suffers—where, when,

What are chills?

When your hypothalamus has received signals to raise your body temperature, you experience chills. Chills are really a fast way to raise body temperature. The quaking of muscles all over your body produces a lot of heat; that's why you shiver in a cold environment. Shivering is one of your body's built-in protective reflexes to restore body heat. Generally, you're not truly cold when fever chills begin, but the hypothalamus has turned on the shivering reflex to push your body temperature upwards. You'll think you're cold because shivering and fever chills are exactly the same sensation.

When the work of your hypothalamus and your immune system is done, your body must dump all the extra heat it has developed. You'll have sweats, the usual sign that a fever has "broken." Just as perspiration cools you by evaporation after heavy exertion, it will restore a lower body temperature after a fever.

and how often. Researchers have found that anyone, anywhere, may catch colds, but some people have more colds than others. Further, colds are seasonal events for some people.

Children catch the most colds, about six each year as infants, tapering off to two or three in adolescence. As you become older, your colds become rarer, one or two each year. (Though if you've become a parent, you're apt to catch a few more colds while your children have them.) Women catch more colds than men; no one knows why. And poor people have colds more frequently than other people.

We call this viral infection a "cold," so we must feel it's related to cold weather. Statistics show we're at least half correct: colds in the United States and other nontropical nations are likeliest to occur in November, December, and January. Millions of colds occur in every month, however, and countries without a cold season record as many colds as more northerly nations. Tropical colds peak in the wetter seasons, though. We, too, catch more colds when our seasons change, about half as many each spring as during the December peak. As far as scientists can now tell, cold viruses don't have any preference for weather, but weather that keeps us indoors may make contagion easier.

Another finding probably won't surprise you: you're more likely to come down with a cold on Monday than on any other day.

The killer cold
We can be confident of recovery from a cold because our immune system contains the knowledge to disarm a wide variety of cold viruses. To a population not previously exposed to colds, these same viruses can be killers. Again and again, history records a tragic sequel to the first meetings of Europeans with inhabitants of South America. Indian populations were decimated, as by a plague, when first infected by the "common cold."

Meaning of "-itis"

In general, any medical word ending in -itis indicates some sort of inflammation. Whatever you put in front of -itis names the affected area. For example, laryngitis *means an inflammation of your vocal cords and surrounding tissue—a larynx inflammation, in other words. Those terms you're most likely to encounter when talking about colds (on medication labels, for example) are* rhinitis *(from Greek* rhino, *"nose"),* sinusitis *(from Latin, meaning* hollow*),* pharyngitis *(from* pharynx, *your upper throat),* tonsillitis, *otitis (from Greek* oto, *"ear"), and* bronchitis *(from* bronchi, *the major air passageways within your lungs).*

How to tell if you have a cold

We're all quite sure we know what we're talking about when we say we have a cold. Usually, we notice first vague feelings of tiredness (fatigue) and achiness, followed by a sore throat, runny nose, slight fever, and sinus congestion. Of course, the symptom list could go on; everyone's cold is a little different. Some colds bring chills, cough, laryngitis, and other symptoms—but even though this symptom list grows confusingly long, we still think we know when we have a cold. Why? Aren't we really describing many different diseases with so many symptoms?

Despite a cold's many guises, we recognize it by several important clues:

—A cold's symptoms generally worsen for the first 4 or 5 days and then improve. We expect a cold to all but disappear within 10 days or 2 weeks at the most.

If your symptoms don't begin to clear within 5 days, you may well have some other disease. By the same token, if low-level symptoms—fatigue, aches, slight fevers—persist beyond 10 to 14 days, you should see a doctor.

—Cold symptoms, though varied, are rarely intense. Fever shouldn't be very high. Any fever as high as 102° F. in adults or 103° F. in children probably indicates an illness other than a cold. Nor is a cold's fever constant.

Sore throat from a cold isn't as painful as that brought on by a bacterial inflammation, such as strep. Watery eyes, runny nose, and congestion, so typical of a cold, can occur also as allergic reactions. But allergy symptoms usually begin quickly, within an hour or two. Cold sufferers usually know they're afflicted a day or two before nasal and sinus congestion appear.

—Despite cold misery variations, some symptoms don't belong: constant headache, earache, a rash, weakness, swollen neck glands, breathing difficulty, or racking cough. These complaints need medical attention. When you experience such symptoms, suspect a disorder other than a cold. Don't try to treat yourself—get a doctor's opinion.

Thus we have three rules of thumb for deciding when we have a cold:

—The symptoms shouldn't last longer than 10 days, with marked improvement after the fourth or fifth day.

—Although several symptoms may be involved, none is painfully intense.

You haven't lost your sense of taste

One of a cold's most familiar miseries is taste loss. But scientists say the problem isn't with taste. Your tongue's sensation isn't much changed during a cold, but your sense of smell diminishes.

Perhaps you've never realized how much your sense of smell adds to your food enjoyment. Aromas move through your nasal cavities even while food is in your mouth. Your smell-sensing nerves respond to stimuli up to 25,000 times weaker than those your taste buds can detect. Thus, without your keen sense of smell, your tongue identifies only the strongest, simplest flavors.

—Constant headache, earache, a rash, weakness, swollen neck glands, breathing difficulty, or racking cough should alert us to look for illnesses other than a cold.

You may still confuse a cold with some other ailment, because several illnesses cause symptoms similar to a cold's. The greatest similarity is between a cold and some types of influenza.

Is it a cold or the flu?

You won't always know whether you have a cold or the flu because the symptoms of the two illnesses can be too much alike. However, as long as the flu behaves like a cold and disappears about as quickly, the answer really isn't important—certainly not worth expensive testing to find out.

Influenza tends to infect more of your body than a cold virus. Influenza becomes more deeply seated in your respiratory tract and often holds on longer. Serious complications, such as pneumonia, can follow influenza, particularly in people whose health is already somewhat impaired. For this reason, public health officials and some doctors recommend preventive flu vaccines for young children and for adults over age 65 or those with chronic disease. Generally, flu vaccines are used by those with a higher health vulnerability to flu complications.

Flu develops suddenly, so you may justly suspect you have flu when your symptoms appear as shortly as an hour after your first hint of illness. In a flu attack, you'll experience more muscle aches than you would with a cold. And your fever will rise higher. A flu fever may reach 102° F. or higher and may drop only to shoot upward several times daily. Chills, too, occur more often with the flu. Lastly, flu's cough is more frequent and more troublesome.

Don't assume that you have a cold just because you're sneezing and have watery eyes and a runny nose. These symptoms belong equally to an influenza infection or an allergic reaction.

Some of flu's details resemble those of a cold, with the exception that flu symptoms intensify more quickly. Both diseases are likely to be with you for 7 to 10 days, peaking at about the fourth or fifth day. What we sometimes refer to as the "24-hour flu"—a quick, intense, usually intestinal infection—is often caused by a virus, but not one related to influenza.

It's a misnamed disease.

See your doctor if your symptoms haven't disappeared in a week to 10 days, if the symptoms are unusually severe, or if you develop abnormal symptoms (breathing difficulty, swollen neck glands, rash, or extremely painful cough). You can read more about flu in Chapter 8.

Avoiding a cold

Commonsense notions about how colds are transmitted stand up fairly well to scientific testing. Coughing and sneezing spread the virus, as does close contact. The details of contagion give us a clearer picture. For instance, cold viruses don't really drift through the air; they're usually carried on minute moisture droplets expelled when someone coughs or sneezes. And although we may stay well clear of a cold sufferer, and beyond sneezing range, we still

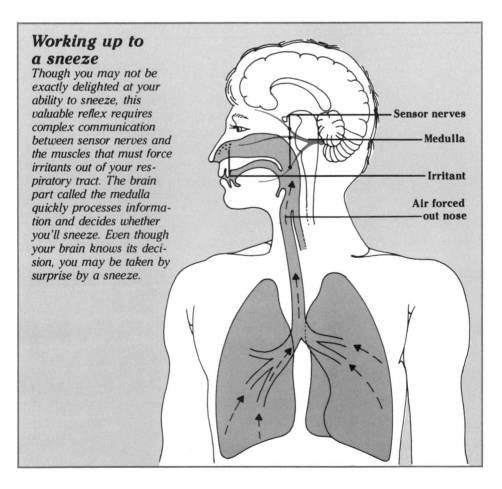

Working up to a sneeze
Though you may not be exactly delighted at your ability to sneeze, this valuable reflex requires complex communication between sensor nerves and the muscles that must force irritants out of your respiratory tract. The brain part called the medulla quickly processes information and decides whether you'll sneeze. Even though your brain knows its decision, you may be taken by surprise by a sneeze.

Sensor nerves

Medulla

Irritant

Air forced out nose

Eye infection—a possible cold complication

Some viruses that cause colds, particularly adenovirus, may infect the lining of your eyelids. Called conjunctivitis, this cold complication will give you uncomfortable lid swelling and a clear discharge from under your lids. The swelling may itch a little. Avoiding conjunctivitis is one very good reason to keep your hands away from your eyes, especially while you or someone else in the family is suffering from a cold. If the discharge from your eye turns cloudy or yellow to greenish, you probably have bacterial conjunctivitis. Your doctor can give you an ointment to soothe your inflamed lids and kill the harmful bacteria.

While you have conjunctivitis, take special care in washing your hands, using clean towels, and not touching your eyes.

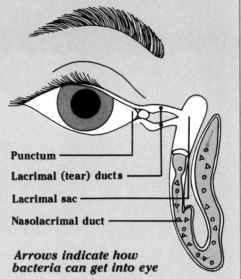

Punctum

Lacrimal (tear) ducts

Lacrimal sac

Nasolacrimal duct

Arrows indicate how bacteria can get into eye

Sinuses

Your sinuses are perhaps more extensive than you thought, and they all must drain into your nasal cavity. Since the sinus openings are quite small, any blockage or excessive mucus will cause the familiar throbbing facial pain of colds sometimes described as a sinus headache.

haven't avoided the chief infection risk: contact with surfaces harboring the still-active virus.

Cold viruses, as a rule, survive poorly outside living tissue, but they cope well enough for a few hours. The average cold sufferer lives temporarily within a cloud of viral particles, originating in the respiratory tract and brought into contact with the skin through breathing, sneezing, nose blowing, and so forth. The hands—from rubbing the eyes, touching the nose, or shielding a cough—constantly carry a viral dose. A quick handshake spreads more infection than the most explosive sneeze.

Two or three days before cold symptoms appear, the victim begins to spread the virus. A cold sufferer remains contagious until symptoms begin to diminish, at the fifth day or later.

Anything a cold victim touches—such as utensils, medication bottles, light switches, telephones, doorknobs—remains a potential infection source for a few hours. How do you catch the cold? After you've handled an infected object, you might rub your eyes, or your nose, and suddenly you're infected.

The eyes and nose, by the way, are the chief viral routes into your body. (You should *always* wash your hands before touching the eyes—as when inserting a contact lens. The eyes have poor immune defenses

Upper airway defenses against infection

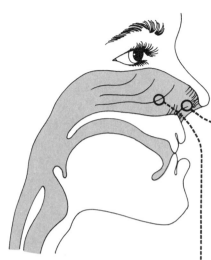

Nasal passage

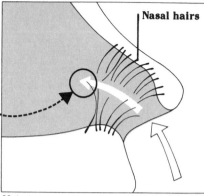

Hair in nose traps dirt, dust, and grit.

The upper airways form the front line in defending the body from infection. Nasal hairs trap dust and large particles when you inhale. Mucus then traps finer particles, which the cilia move to the oropharynx (mouth area) for swallowing. At the same time, turbinates—bony structures that project into the nasal cavity—humidify and warm the air, which keeps secretions moist and loose. In the pharynx, the soft palate and epiglottis separate air and food, preventing choking. The gag and cough reflexes also prevent choking, and the cough reflex clears secretions that might provide a medium for bacterial growth.

Turbinates

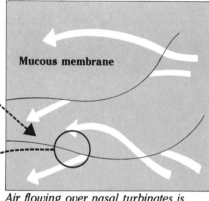

Air flowing over nasal turbinates is warmed and moistened.

Microscopic view of turbinates

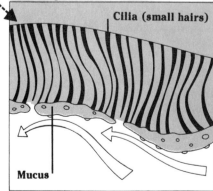

Small hairs (cilia) and mucus trap small particles not caught by nasal hairs.

Epiglottitis

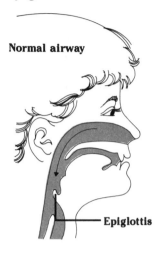

Normal airway

Epiglottis

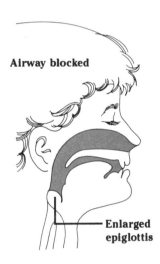

Airway blocked

Enlarged epiglottis

Though not very common, epiglottis infection can happen, particularly in children between ages 2 and 5. Infections that may turn into epiglottitis start with sudden fever, sore throat, and hoarseness. At the first signs of suspected epiglottitis—difficulty swallowing, drooling, and rapid, gasping breaths—take the victim to an emergency room.

and make a perfect entryway for many infections.) Strangely, picking up a cold virus through your mouth isn't very likely. No one knows why; perhaps the mouth's chemistry doesn't suit cold viruses.

These findings about cold contagion affirm general hygienic principles. Wash your hands frequently, avoid rubbing your eyes, clean much-used surfaces (such as doorknobs, telephones, utensils), and dispose of heavily contaminated materials (such as used tissues). You may still catch a cold, though, even after you've done as much as you sensibly can to avoid it.

Your respiratory tract

To understand what happens to your body when a cold virus invades, you'll want to understand your respiratory tract. The respiratory tract includes everything along the route that air takes to reach your lungs, from your nose to the branching bronchi and bronchioles that divide the incoming airstream and distribute it within the lungs themselves.

—Turbinates. The empty spaces immediately behind your nose contain long, bony scrolls called the turbinates. The turbinates warm and channel the air you breathe. From the turbinates all the way into the lungs, air is in contact with mucus-lined tissue. Mucus removes a great deal of air dust and particles, including a good percentage of the microbes you inhale. These mucous tissues also contain millions of invisible small hairs (about half a thousandth inch long) called cilia. Cilia are always waving gently—moving mucus slowly to the throat for ultimate ingestion by the stomach.

—Sinuses. Your sinus cavities help to provide more mucus for the turbinates and nostrils. These empty chambers in your face's bony structure produce mucus that prevents your nostrils from becoming dry and painful. If mucus doesn't drain properly from your sinuses, you'll experience discomfort. As you must have noticed, especially when your sinuses are clogged, they work as sound resonators, adding certain qualities to your voice.

—Pharynx. From the back of your nasal cavity to the beginning of your main airway (the trachea), air travels through the pharynx—the same pathway taken by food on its way to the esophagus—and down into your lungs. Since this part of your respiratory tract serves both your mouth and nose, you can still breathe when one or the other is blocked—a supreme advantage. But an occasional food particle or sip of

Cold sores

Sometime during a cold's course, you may notice blisterlike sores on your lips or mouth—cold sores. These eruptions have little to do with colds; they're caused by a different virus altogether, herpes simplex type 1.

By age 6 or 7, practically everyone has been exposed to herpes simplex, usually in the form of chicken pox but sometimes without symptoms. Though scientists still have many unanswered questions about herpes simplex, researchers believe this organism resides permanently in certain nerve tissue, including that around the mouth. Many kinds of irritation and stress, both physical and psychological, may cause an outbreak.

You can't cure a cold sore. Until the sore forms a crusty scab, after 4 or 5 days, the fluid inside it contains an active virus. In the meantime, wash the affected area and your hands to minimize the chances of transmitting the infection to other parts of your body or to others.

liquid destined for the stomach can find its way into your windpipe, causing coughing.

—Adenoids and tonsils. Located in your throat at the very back of the mouth are your tonsils, one on either side of the tongue's base. Above them and out of sight behind the roof of your mouth are the adenoids. Adenoids and tonsils are somewhat mystifying. Because they seemed to do nothing but swell painfully during childhood infections, doctors for many years favored surgical removal of tonsils and adenoids at an early age. We know now that these glands are a working part of the body's immune system. You may think of them as reservoirs holding a supply of specialized, infection-fighting cells.

—Epiglottis. Keeping food out of your lungs when you swallow is the job of your epiglottis. This stiff flap, located behind and below the tongue, automatically folds backward when you swallow and seals off the trachea. When food passes it, your epiglottis springs upward, restoring free air passage into your windpipe. The epiglottis plays no direct role in fighting disease, but is crucial to your coughing obstructions or congestion out of your airway.

—Larynx. Your windpipe's entryway, where your vocal cords are located, is called the larynx. Softer tissue than the trachea, the larynx also hosts more infections. (Not all larynx inflammations—laryngitis—are caused by infection; straining your voice may also cause irritation.)

Beyond the larynx lies the rest of your respiratory tract. Pretty much all of it can host an infection—and it's exposed with your every breath to microscopic organisms. The fact that we suffer only infrequently from serious infection proves the effectiveness of our defenses.

4

What to Do about Your Cold

Once you've decided you have a cold, your wisest course mixes rest, a sensible diet, and perhaps a few medications with alertness for symptoms that may signal more serious health complications.

Rest

No prescription is more valuable for the average cold than a few days of rest. You don't have to take to your bed, but you should reduce your activities—a good time to read, write letters, watch television. You'll notice that your energy level will change widely during the day. When your weariness increases, when aches interfere with your concentration, don't fight it. Rest.

Taking a day or two off work is a good idea—not that you'll spare your co-workers exposure to your infection, for they've already had that. However, the less you strain yourself during your cold, the milder your symptoms are apt to be. And, anyway, no one works very efficiently with a pounding head, runny nose, and slight fever.

Taking the best possible care of yourself may not make your cold go away sooner. However, you'll feel less miserable and probably suffer fewer complications.

Diet

No special menu will help relieve your cold symptoms. Eat whatever you find appetizing. The often-heard advice, "Feed a cold, starve a fever," can't hurt you but really only makes medical sense for people with high fevers or an intestinal disease—their stomachs may reject all but the blandest food.

Warm fluids, such as tea or soup, help break up congestion (warm vapors seem to speed up mucous flow) and are worth a try. In general, though, the best dietary advice to a cold sufferer is just to keep up good nutrition.

Treating symptoms

The most irritating cold symptoms are usually some combination of sore throat, cough, sinus congestion, runny nose, headache, and slight fever with muscle aches. The prominence of one kind of symptom over

Cold or warm mist: Which is best?

Vaporizers, which make steam, and humidifiers, which produce minute water droplets, will both do a satisfactory job of keeping the air around you moist. Both need a certain amount of care (see below). If your primary interest is in loosening up a cold's congestion, you would probably opt for a vaporizer's warm moisture. To keep your home prop-erly humidified, however, particularly if you have a very dry winter heat source, you'll probably want a humidifier, which is cheaper to operate than a vaporizer.

You'll need to clean and disinfect a humidifier from time to time, or mi-crobes will begin to thrive in its cool water. The manufacturer's in-structions will tell you how and when to clean your humidifier.

Vaporizer operation builds mineral deposits (scale) around the heat-ing element. You must re-move these deposits periodically with vinegar or other cleaners (usually specified in your vapor-izer instructions). If you let the scale build up, the heating coils will work less and less efficiently, leading to low steam out-put or burned-out coils.

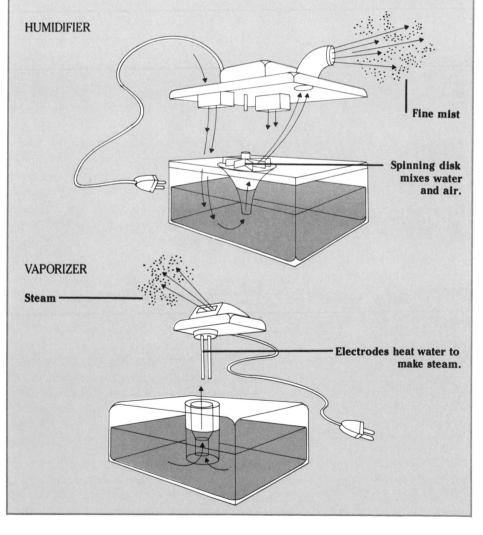

HUMIDIFIER

Fine mist

Spinning disk mixes water and air.

VAPORIZER

Steam

Electrodes heat water to make steam.

Alcohol and medication—often a mistake

The list of drugs that can be dangerous when taken with alcoholic drinks is a long one—including most medications that have a sedative or slowing effect on your body. As far as common cold remedies are concerned, you'd be wise to avoid drinking any alcoholic beverages within 6 to 8 hours of taking antihistamines, decongestants, or codeine. Alcohol doesn't merely add to a medication's sedative power but actually multiplies this side effect.

the others often leads us to characterize a cold as "loose" or "tight," as a "head cold" or "chest cold," but medically a cold's a cold. We'll examine each of these symptoms in turn and suggest ways to lessen their discomfort.

Sore throat

Throat tissue inflammation is a cold's hallmark. All the viruses that collectively may cause what we loosely term a cold strongly favor your throat as an infection site. What you can do about a sore throat doesn't promise dramatic relief but can help.

Gargling with warm salt water (something that singers and speakers with strained, scratchy throats also do) can soothe your throat. Throat lozenges, dissolved slowly in the mouth, coat the whole throat passage but usually bring only limited relief for soreness. Many OTC products contain active anesthetic ingredients, but the FDA finds that the dosage levels in such products aren't high enough to be effective.

In all cases, discontinue throat irritants, such as cigarettes, at least for the duration of your sore throat or cough.

Cough

Your cold's cough rarely needs attention. If the cough is a productive one, you won't wish to interfere. If, on the other hand, you have a ticklish, dry cough, you can try coating your throat. Dissolve a little honey in tea and sip slowly, or suck on a piece of hard candy. (Diabetics, however, can't look to any sugary or alcohol-containing remedy.)

Sinus congestion

When mucus drains too slowly from inflamed sinuses, the throbbing result is the classic stuffiness of a cold. You can speed up the draining process by inhaling warm vapors. Plain steam works as well as anything else. Standing in a steamy shower or holding your toweled head over a steaming water basin may bring some relief. Don't inhale really hot steam; you could injure your respiratory tract tissues. You might wish, also, to moisten the air around you with a vaporizer or humidifier. The moister the air you breathe, the easier mucus moves through swollen sinus passages.

Runny nose

Everyone has a personal technique for coping with a runny nose. Some techniques are wiser than others, however. Forceful nose blowing, especially while clos-

How to use a nasal spray

1. Before you begin, read the medication label carefully, so you know the exact amount of the spray to administer. Make sure you have tissues or a handkerchief handy. Then, sit upright, with your head tilted back.

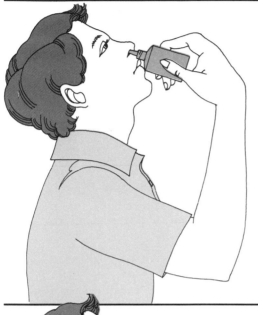

2. Place the tip of the squeeze bottle about ½ inch inside your nostril. Point it straight up your nose, as though you were aiming for your eye's inner corner. Don't angle the squeeze bottle downward, or the medication will run down your throat.

Without inhaling, squeeze the bottle once, quickly and firmly. Use just enough force to coat the inside of your nose with medication. Then, spray again if the instructions on the label order it. Repeat the procedure in the other nostril.

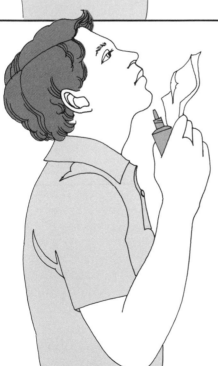

3. Keep your head tilted back for several minutes, so the medication has time to work. (If you lower your head, the medication will drain out your nose—not what you want.) Don't blow your nose while you wait.

Reye's syndrome

Reye's syndrome is an extremely seri-ous complication, usually seen in chil-dren under age 18, that can follow chicken pox, measles, flu, and a few other viral infections. Though rare, this complication can result in liver changes, brain swelling, heart damage, coma, and death. It occurs in children from infancy to adolescence, and recent stud-ies show that it occurs more frequently in children who have been given aspirin for their viral fevers.

Aspirin labels now warn that children who may be suffering from flu, mea-sles, or chicken pox should not be given aspirin. You may try an aspirin substi-tute, such as acetaminophen, if you wish, or call your doctor for advice if your child is running a high fever.

If your child is ill and shows signs of confusion, lethargy, seizures, or diffi-culty breathing, take the child immedi-ately to a hospital for treatment. Tell the doctor you have observed signs that lead you to suspect Reye's syndrome.

WARNING: Children and teenagers should not use this medicine for chicken pox or flu symptoms before a doctor is consulted about Reye's syndrome, a rare but serious illness.

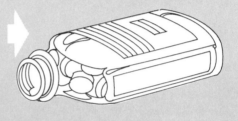

ing off one of your nostrils, builds pressure. You could force mucus back into your sinus passages or through your eustachian tube into your ear. In fact, you could set up an infection in your middle ear. Blow, if you must, but blow gently, simultaneously through both nostrils, and into a disposable tissue.

Frequent nose blowing may irritate the tip of your nose, causing chafing and chapping. You can alleviate this raw discomfort by applying petroleum jelly to reddened skin, preferably every hour or so.

Headache, fever, muscle aches

A cold's fever seldom lasts very long, nor is it severe. (If your fever persists, or climbs above 102° F., see a doctor; that symptom suggests something other than a cold.) To treat your feverish aches and pound-ing head, try aspirin. If aspirin's side effects make it a poor choice for you, try acetaminophen. Neither of these common drugs can cure your cold, but both may reduce your discomfort.

Some medical philosophy about colds

If you're in good health, a cold isn't a medical crisis, and you can go overboard trying to treat it. In general, the stronger the drugs you use to treat a cold's symp-

Cold carriers

Any nonabsorbent surface that receives a lot of com-mon use by family mem-bers is a likely source of cold contamination. But the most contaminated surfaces are likely to be your hands. That's why you should wash them fre-quently during the day, whether you're around a cold sufferer or not.

Caution with decongestants

Carefully read the ingredients and manufacturer's warnings on any decongestant, particularly an oral decongestant. Frequently, one active ingredient is a close relative to the drugs used in bronchodilators for asthma relief; such ingredients include ephedrine, epinephrine, and albuterol. Consequently, user cautions are very much alike—don't use a decongestant if you suffer from high blood pressure, heart disease, or thyroid disease. Other warnings may apply to specific OTC products. Some medications may not be safe for people taking MAO inhibitors or suffering from asthma, glaucoma, diabetes, or prostate disease.

toms, the more effectively you might mask a more serious illness—a strep infection, for example. When symptoms persist, of course, you'll suspect something other than a cold, but you'll have lost valuable time.

Do what you can for your cold, but don't use unnecessary medications. If you aren't getting any better after 4 or 5 days, take careful note of your symptoms and read Chapter 5. You may need medical help.

Decongestants, antihistamines, and other cold drugs

Most OTC cold medications contain a decongestant, an antihistamine, or an analgesic (a mild pain reliever, such as aspirin), or any combination of the three. All three will give you some relief for cold symptoms: antihistamines will dry up mucus; decongestants shrink swollen membranes; and analgesics soothe your aches. Preferably, buy one product to do one thing at a time. Antihistamines probably work better for allergies like hay fever than for colds. Decongestants are fine for colds, but you shouldn't take them by mouth if you have high blood pressure, hyperthyroidism, or take monoamine oxidase (MAO) inhibitors for depression.

Decongestants needn't be taken by mouth. You can select from nose sprays, nose drops, and inhalants. Don't exceed the manufacturer's recommended dosages, and don't use a decongestant for more than a few days. One decongestant side effect from overuse

Treating yourself right

Select medications with these points in mind:
• *Treat one symptom at a time. Medications with a long list of active ingredients to counteract many symptoms rarely work well. Some compound formulations actually make no sense, trying, for example, to dry up congestion and to thin it for easier flow at the same time.*
• *Don't take medications prescribed for other illnesses. Antibiotics, anti-inflammatory drugs, or painkillers that may have been prescribed for past illnesses may cause unwelcome complications. At*
the very least, you may succeed in masking your symptoms.
• *Don't try to suppress a productive cough. See a doctor if it doesn't go away in a week to 10 days.*
• *Don't give aspirin to children who may have viral diseases such as chicken pox, measles, or flu.*
• *With the average cough or cold, you can achieve about the same amount of symptomatic relief with home remedies as with OTC products. Gargles, vaporizers, warm fluids, and soothing syrups work as well as anything else.*

Giving nose drops

To instill nose drops properly, follow these steps.

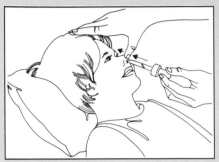

1. Open the person's nostril by pushing up gently on the tip of the nose.

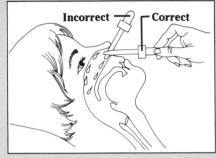

2. Place the dropper about ⅓ inch inside the nose. Direct the dropper upward toward the person's eye. Then squeeze the bulb to instill the correct number of drops.

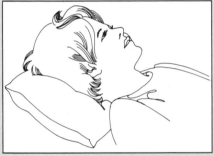

3. The person must keep his head tilted back for about 5 minutes.

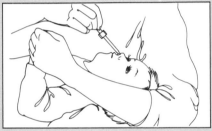

4. If the person is a young child, place him on his back with a small pillow under his shoulders. Tilt his head back, holding it against your arm.

is *increased* congestion.

If you're thinking about taking something for the cough that came with your cold, first read about coughs and OTC cough medications in Chapter 10.

A word about aspirin

Because aspirin is so widely and safely used, you may not think twice about taking a few tablets for a cold's fever, aches, and pains. But aspirin can have side effects, too, just like other drugs. You should know what to look for.

Ringing in the ears or a drop in hearing may be the first aspirin sensitivity sign. A full-scale allergic reaction, with rash or breathing difficulties, indicates a serious aspirin sensitivity. Too much aspirin, even

Chicken soup works
Drinking hot fluids is one of the best ways to relieve nasal congestion. The steamy vapors speed up mucus flow, though only for a half hour or so. And if you're thinking about filling up a thermos with something hot and steamy, you can do no better than hot chicken soup. This particular hot fluid works as well as or better than others tested to break up congestion. It's low in calories, so you may drink it as often as you wish to take advantage of its sinus-clearing powers.

Aspirin's effects on your blood
Aspirin is sometimes used for an effect other than to reduce pain or fever: as an anticoagulant. (Aspirin slows blood clotting.) For this reason, some medical authorities recommend aspirin for people with an increased risk of stroke (caused by a blood clot in the brain). But anticoagulant effects aren't desirable for everyone, especially for persons exposed to a risk of bleeding. Pregnant women, hemophiliacs, or anyone who has had or will soon have surgery should avoid aspirin.

for people who aren't allergic, can cause some bleeding, and pain, in the stomach. Try to take aspirin with meals to minimize any stomach irritation. If aspirin gives you troublesome symptoms, try another pain-killer, such as acetaminophen.

Aspirin labels warn against giving aspirin to a child who may have flu, measles, or chicken pox. Some research links aspirin to a severe flu complication called Reye's syndrome. Follow the manufacturer's caution.

What not to do for a cold

Denying to yourself that you have a cold makes little sense. Once a virus has invaded your body, symptoms inevitably follow. What viruses do produces a certain response from your immune system. In spite of these truths, some people do strange things for a cold. Here's a partial list of popular cold treatments, ranging from magical to foolish and even to dangerous. How many of these have you tried?

Pretend not to notice early symptoms, and they'll go away. Sure, most colds are slight infections, disappearing after as little as a day of congestion or vague aches. Ignoring your symptoms, though, doesn't discourage or dishearten the virus. Factors that determine your vulnerability are extremely complex—and usually beyond your control. You cannot, for instance, choose which of the hundreds of eligible viruses you'll host. Nor do you have the opportunity to pick a best time, to schedule your infection like a dental appointment.

Sweat and physically exhaust yourself, and the virus will disappear. This is a strategy for self-destruction. Coping with viral (or bacterial) invaders makes large demands on your body. Your tissues are clearing themselves of toxic by-products, trying to neutralize viruses, and beginning repairs to damaged areas. The heart carries an extra load in maintaining body temperature; other organs—even those not actually near infected sites—assist in your overall immunologic response. And yet some misguided sufferers believe heavy physical activity will speed up their recovery. What usually happens, of course, is not a normal recovery but a lingering illness.

Heavy exertion during an infection can have a graver result: if you've misdiagnosed yourself—par-

(continued on page 43)

Nonprescription medications for cold symptoms

You can treat your separate cold and cough symptoms with medications available over the counter (but always read and heed the manufacturer's instructions and warnings).

Symptom	Medication
Aches and pains	Aspirin or acetaminophen
Chapping around nose or lips	Petroleum jelly
Congestion (allergy or colds)	*Decongestants:* Active ingredients may include ephedrine, pseudoephedrine, oxymetazoline, naphazoline, or phenylephrine, among others.
Cough, nonproductive	*Anesthetic* ingredients include phenol and benzocaine; *suppressant* ingredients include codeine, dextromethorphan, and benzonatate; *demulcents* (to soothe and coat irritated tissue) include a wide range of syrups and lozenges.
Cough, productive	(Don't suppress a productive cough.) *Expectorants:* Loosen and enhance a productive cough with active ingredients such as terpin hydrate, guaifenesin, ammonium chloride, sodium citrate, or menthol. The FDA has found no expectorant effective; warm fluids and steam work equally well.
Fever	Aspirin or acetaminophen
Runny nose (allergy)	*Antihistamines:* Active ingredients may include diphenhydramine, brompheniramine, chlorpheniramine, or doxylamine, among others.

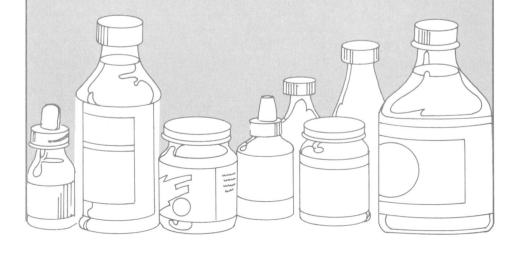

What nonprescription cold medications contain

Most nonprescription cold products combine a decongestant and an antihistamine—and sometimes an analgesic. If you have an adverse reaction, you can try another that doesn't have the same ingredients. Use this chart to guide you.

TABLETS AND CAPSULES

Product	Decongestant	Antihistamine	Analgesic
Actifed tablets and capsules	pseudoephedrine	triprolidine	—
Alka-Seltzer Plus Cold Medicine tablets	phenylpropanolamine	chlorpheniramine	aspirin
Allerest Headache Strength Tablets	phenylpropanolamine	chlorpheniramine	acetaminophen
Allerest Tablets	phenylpropanolamine	chlorpheniramine	—
Benadryl Decongestant Capsules	pseudoephedrine	diphenhydramine	—
Chlor-Trimeton Decongestant Tablets	pseudoephedrine	chlorpheniramine	—
Codimal capsules and tablets	pseudoephedrine	chlorpheniramine	acetaminophen
Contac Capsules	phenylpropanolamine	chlorpheniramine	—
Coricidin 'D' Decongestant Tablets	phenylpropanolamine	chlorpheniramine	acetaminophen
Coricidin Tablets	—	chlorpheniramine	acetaminophen
Dimetane Decongestant Tablets	phenylephrine	brompheniramine	—
Dimetapp Tablets	phenylpropanolamine	brompheniramine	—
Dristan Advanced Formula capsules and tablets	phenylephrine phenylpropanolamine	chlorpheniramine	acetaminophen
Dristan 12-Hour Nasal Decongestant Capsules	phenylephrine	chlorpheniramine	—
Drixoral Tablets	pseudoephedrine	dexbrompheniramine	—
4-Way Cold Tablets	phenylpropanolamine	chlorpheniramine	aspirin

(continued)

What nonprescription cold medications contain *(continued)*

Product	Decongestant	Antihistamine	Analgesic
Ornex Capsules	phenylpropanolamine	—	acetaminophen
Sine-Off Tablets	phenylpropanolamine	chlorpheniramine	aspirin
Teldrin Multi-Symptom Allergy Reliever Capsules	pseudoephedrine	chlorpheniramine	acetaminophen
Triaminic Cold Tablets	phenylpropanolamine	chlorpheniramine	—
Triaminicin Tablets	phenylpropanolamine	chlorpheniramine	aspirin, caffeine

NOSE DROPS AND SPRAYS

Product	Ingredient	Percentage in drops	Percentage in spray
Afrin	oxymetazoline	0.025%, 0.05%	0.05%
Alconefrin	phenylephrine	0.16%, 0.25%, 0.5%	0.25%
Coricidin Nasal Mist	phenylephrine	—	0.5%
Duration	oxymetazoline	—	0.05%
Neo-Synephrine	phenylephrine	0.125%, 0.25%, 0.5%, 1%	0.25%, 0.5%
Neo-Synephrine 12 Hour, Children's	oxymetazoline	0.05%	—
Nōstril	phenylephrine	—	0.25% (pump spray), 0.5%
NTZ Long Acting	oxymetazoline	0.05%	0.05%
Otrivin	xylometazoline	0.05%, 0.1%	0.1%
Privine	naphazoline	0.05%	0.05%
Sinex	phenylephrine	—	0.5%
Sinex Long-Acting	oxymetazoline	—	0.05%

Colds don't cause inflamed tonsils

If your tonsils are painful, swollen, and reddened, like those shown here, you may be suffering from a bacterial infection. See a doctor.

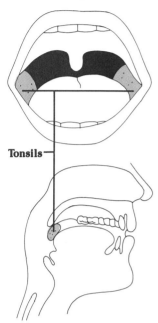

Tonsils

ticularly if you have a bacterial disease—you run the risk of creating secondary infections in those organs you stress most during exercise—the heart and lungs. Don't take this risk; don't exert yourself when you're sick. If you're lucky, your attempt to "sweat out" or "work off" an infection will just make you a little more miserable for a little longer. If you're less lucky, you'll cause serious complications.

Obliterate your symptoms with alcohol—at least you won't suffer. This is the reasoning behind many cold "cures" that rely mostly on alcohol's effects. Relieving symptoms may well be the only real treatment for colds, but use good judgment. Alcohol in large doses brings its own special misery; it places another load on your body. In addition, alcohol often has an unwanted additive effect when taken with other kinds of medication. You may unwittingly multiply the strength of other remedies, or magnify unwanted side effects.

Even when taken by itself, an alcoholic preparation—for example, a hot toddy or mulled wine—will merely add to such common cold symptoms as congestion and headache. Spare yourself the added misery.

Take every medicine you can lay your hands on—something's bound to work. This is sometimes called the "shotgun" approach to curing a cold. Maybe if a cold were a rare and life-threatening disease, such measures could be justified. But colds come and go, usually doing little health damage. They don't warrant a dangerous drug mix.

Perhaps an impatient cold sufferer's chief medication abuse involves drugs prescribed for other purposes entirely that are still on the medicine shelf. Strong painkillers and antibiotics aren't for colds. Don't invite troublesome results by taking inappropriate medications.

Another temptation for cold sufferers is to relieve all cold symptoms at once. Some OTC products have more ingredients than are effective. A product claiming to handle all symptoms—pain, cough, congestion, sore throat, runny nose, and fever—can't deliver what it promises, but it will be more expensive.

FDA studies have confirmed that otherwise proven ingredients may not work if the dosage is too small. In other words, you may be wasting your money when you buy a product for its collection of ingredients.

5 When Can Your Doctor Help?

Croup
One complication that isn't brought on by invading bacteria is croup. Usually, croup appears only in children age 3 or under, but older children and adults occasionally get it. You'll recognize croup by the distinctive, barking cough that announces it. For a fuller description of croup and what to do about it, see Chapter 10.

Complications can add to your cold miseries, especially bronchitis, earache, or sinusitis. You'll want a doctor's help for such complications.

Bronchitis

During a cold, bronchitis appears first as a hacking cough and sore throat. Your temperature may rise to 101° to 102° F. The cough becomes more productive, bringing up mucus, within a day or two. What these symptoms mean is that your throat or deeper airways have become infected, sometimes by bacteria taking advantage of viral damage. Often, when you say that a cold moves into your chest, you're describing the onset of bronchitis.

Normally, bronchitis disappears in 3 or 4 days. If your symptoms don't seem to clear up, or if they worsen, see a doctor—bronchitis can lead to pneumonia. If you suffer from a chronic heart or lung disease, see your doctor as soon as you suspect you have bronchitis.

Earache

Bacteria may also travel through your eustachian tube to your ear, where they cause a painful earache (otitis media). The eustachian tube is a short canal running from inside your ear to the upper throat. Bacteria that reach the middle ear greatly worsen the ear's inflammation (usually, virus is already active there). As fluids build up, putting pressure on the eardrum, pain can be excruciating. Ear infections can rob you of hearing or attack bones around the ear. Dizziness, sudden profound hearing loss, or chills and high fever are serious symptoms during an earache. See a doctor for pain relief and for antibiotics to handle the infection.

Sinusitis

Occasionally, bacteria move into the sinuses during a viral inflammation. The result is a true sinus infection, sinusitis. Continuing pain or pressure above the eye, in the temples, or in the area around an ear should lead you to suspect sinusitis. Especially typical is pain or pressure that worsens when you sit, move your head forward or to one side, or lie down. Some-

Bronchitis

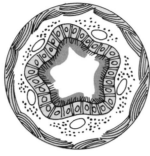

Cross section of normal breathing tube (bronchi)

Narrowed bronchi in bronchitis

Often developing after a cold or other respiratory viral infection, bronchitis is an acute inflammation of the bronchial tubes, which lead from the windpipe to the lungs. Though usually mild and self-limiting, acute bronchitis can be serious, especially in persons with respiratory or cardiac problems. Bacterial infection may complicate bronchitis; untreated bacterial bronchitis can develop into pneumonia.

Early signs and symptoms of bronchitis mimic those of a cold or flu: slight fever, chills, chest discomfort, sore throat, and dry cough. As bronchitis worsens, coughing produces thick mucus, sometimes tinged with blood, and breathing becomes progressively more difficult.

Treatment of uncomplicated bronchitis consists of rest, increased fluid intake, and aspirin or acetaminophen for fever and pain. Symptoms usually subside in 2 to 3 days, although coughing may last for 2 to 3 weeks. Persistent fever may signal developing pneumonia. Call your doctor if symptoms are severe or persist beyond a week; he may prescribe antibiotics.

times the sinusitis pain may even be confused with a toothache—you might feel it as an upper jaw throbbing. See your doctor about any suspected case of sinusitis; this infection can be stubborn and usually requires antibiotics.

Antibiotics

On the manufacturer's information sheet that comes with any antibiotic, you can read about the possible side effects from that particular drug. Or you can read the same information in any comprehensive prescription drug book. As you'll see, antibiotics aren't for casual use. Some antibiotics work against a short list of bacteria; some have broader effectiveness. None destroys viruses. And all have a potential for unpleasant or even serious side effects. A more general antibiotic side effect, however, should discourage you from using borrowed or leftover antibiotics to treat your cold.

Pneumonia

One of the most serious complications of colds and flu, pneumonia usually occurs in one of two forms—bacterial or viral. Bacterial pneumonia, *the most common form*, results from inflammation of lung tissue by any one of several bacteria. It's often caused by seepage of bacteria-laden mucus into the lungs. This can happen if flu viruses damage the cilia that line the respiratory tract and normally help keep mucus out of the lungs. The bacteria in mucus are ordinarily harmless but become highly dangerous when they accumulate in the lungs. Before the development of anti-biotic drugs, the resulting infection was invariably fatal. Even today, with a wide range of antibiotics available, bacterial pneumonia is fatal in about 25% of cases.

How can you recognize the early signs and symptoms of bacterial pneumonia? Like flu, bacterial pneumonia typically causes high fever, chills, chest pain, and coughing. Fever can be quite high—up to 105° or 106° F. Unlike the thin, watery mucus that accompanies flu, the cough in bacterial pneumonia produces a thick yellow or greenish mucus that may contain traces of blood. As pneumonia worsens, breathing becomes more difficult and rapid; pulse rate also quickens. In severe cases, cyanosis—a sign of insufficient oxygen marked by a faint blue tinge under the fingernails or on the lips, ears, and cheeks—may develop.

Viral pneumonia, *the rarest and most deadly form of pneumonia*, results from the spread of flu virus into the lungs. Only about half of the patients with viral pneumonia survive; the death rate is so high because, unlike bacterial pneumonia, viral pneumonia can't be treated with antibiotics, and effective antiviral drugs are still in experimental stages.

Viral pneumonia typically behaves like a serious case of the flu, with rapid onset of high fever, shaking chills, chest pain, headache, severe cough producing thick mucus, and marked cyanosis. Prompt treatment—oxygen, mechanical respiration, and other supportive measures—is necessary to prevent death from respiratory or cardiac collapse.

NORMAL X-RAY

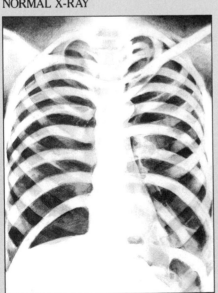

X-RAY INDICATING PNEUMONIA

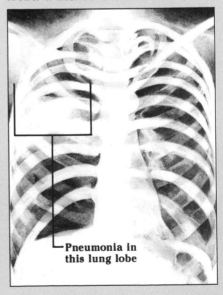

Pneumonia in this lung lobe

Pulmonary function tests

If your doctor suspects that you may have an underlying lung disease, he may ask you to have a pulmonary function test. During this painless test, you'll breathe into a mouthpiece that's attached to a spirometer. This device measures how much air your lungs can hold, how well air moves in and out of your lungs, and how much air remains in your lungs after you exhale normally.

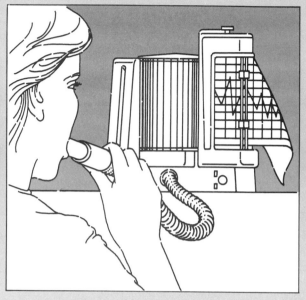

Pneumonia—a potential killer

Pneumonia is a lung infection; colds aren't. Bacteria, viruses, fungi, and other agents cause pneumonia— a very serious disease. So-called double pneumonia isn't a medical term, though doctors once used it to describe pneumonia affecting both lungs.

If you or anyone under your care develops high fever (103° F. or over), chest pain, productive cough with rust-colored sputum, breathing difficulty, and shaking chills—the classic symptoms of pneumonia— get medical treatment immediately.

Just as you wouldn't want to fix something that isn't broken, you won't want to take antibiotics for an infection you don't have. The many bacteria that inhabit a healthy body tend to live in a delicate balance, various species holding each other in check. Antibiotics may selectively wipe out one bacterial species, creating an unwelcome opportunity for another microorganism to flourish, particularly right after you stop taking an antibiotic. This describes a "rebound," or secondary, infection.

You risk a follow-up infection when your body's defenses have been weakened by a virus, whether or not you've taken antibiotics. Your doctor can best decide if you're threatened by possible follow-up bacterial infections and need a preventive dose of a particular antibiotic.

Vaccines

Although colds usually aren't serious illnesses, many of us would just as soon do without them. Besides, a cold can pose a greater health threat to someone suffering from chronic heart or lung disease. Other viral infections like flu respond to vaccines. Why don't we have a cold vaccine?

(continued on page 50)

Vaccination questions and answers

Should I be immunized?
Only your doctor can tell you if you're apt to benefit from a particular flu vaccine. Depending on the specific flu virus and the risk of pandemic, he probably will recommend a flu vaccination if you fall into one of the following high-risk categories:
• persons over age 65
• persons with chronic lung diseases such as asthma, emphysema, chronic bronchitis, tuberculosis, and cystic fibrosis
• persons with heart disease, kidney disease, diabetes, or severe anemia
• persons suffering from cancer or taking a drug that interferes with the body's immune system
• persons who run a high risk of exposure to flu virus, such as health care workers and military personnel
• pregnant women due to deliver in the winter months.

Immunization, preferably done in the fall, usually consists of one dose of vaccine (unless it's for a new flu virus strain, in which case immunization should consist of two vaccinations given 1 month apart). Immunity develops about 2 weeks after vaccination. Because each vaccination provides immunity for 1 to 2 years only, you'll need an annual booster shot for optimal protection.

What about reactions?
Most people have little or no reaction to immunization. About 1 person in 10 will develop slight tenderness, swelling, or redness around the injection site; about 1 in 100 will experience mild fever and headache for a day or two. Of course, if you develop more severe symptoms, you should contact your doctor. Contrary to popular belief, these reactions aren't effects of flu infection; vaccines contain only dead flu virus, which can't infect body tissue. What happens is this: the body's immune system sometimes reacts to dead flu virus as it does to live, infectious virus, causing similar symptoms. The result isn't really flu, although it may feel like flu.

An extremely rare reaction to vaccination was noted during the 1976 swine flu immunization program. Guillain-Barré syndrome, rapidly progressive muscle weakness that results in temporary paralysis, affected about 1 in 100,000 persons vaccinated during the 1976 program; most affected persons recovered completely. Although Guillain-Barré syndrome (which is more commonly associated with natural exposure to a virus) hasn't been seen as a reaction to immunization since the 1976 program, your doctor may still warn you of its remote risk.

What precautions should I take?
Ask your doctor about risks and possible side effects before you get your shot. Also tell him of any allergies you have now or have had. (Many vaccines are prepared in cultures made from chicken eggs and can be dangerous to persons with an allergy to egg proteins. Generally, a vaccine serum cultured in another medium—one that's less likely to produce an allergic reaction—will be available.) And, finally, inform your doctor if you have any kind of infection or have been inoculated for something else within the past few weeks; he may want to postpone your flu vaccination for a few days.

Remember, although reactions do occur in any immunization program, the risk is quite small. Compared to the possible consequences of flu, vaccination—especially for high-risk persons—is almost always the best and safest option.

Understanding vaccines

All vaccines have the same purpose: to give your immune system a safe viral model against which to prepare effective antibodies. Scientists have invented three kinds of vaccines, each challenging the immune system in slightly different ways.

Killed virus vaccines contain viruses that have been completely neutralized; their crucial protein tools for entering cells have been chemically destroyed or plugged up. Enough of the virus is unaltered to allow your immune system to recognize and attack it.

Weakened virus vaccines use whole viruses that have been bred to become fragile. That is, whenever possible, a tough virus (such as polio) that attacks throughout the body is altered to eliminate its chances of survival except in perhaps your nasal membranes. A weakened virus can't spread like its hardier original strain, but it excites your immune system to produce antibodies effective against the whole viral type.

Split virus vaccines contain only parts of a virus—usually parts of the viral outer coat. This is enough to provoke an effective response from your immune system. Split virus vaccines may cause slightly fewer side effects than killed and weakened virus vaccines.

Making vaccines using eggs

In a sterile environment, technicians withdraw virus-laden fluid from inside eggs where the virus was grown. The virus is then filtered from the fluid and made into vaccine. After you get a vaccine (for example, a flu shot), your body is stimulated to produce antibodies against that virus.

Because many vaccines are developed using egg cultures, people who are allergic to egg protein may have an allergic reaction to vaccines. In most cases, a vaccine cultured in another medium will be less likely to produce a reaction.

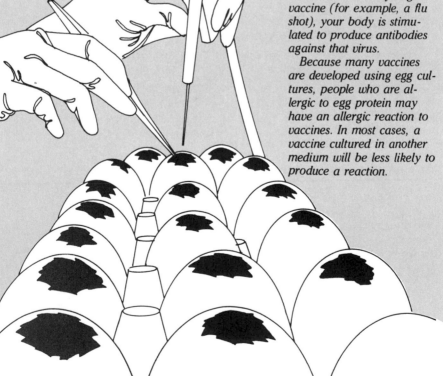

Amantadine

Because viruses work so intimately with the life processes of cells, many scientists thought that any drug that killed viruses would destroy an unacceptable number of healthy cells. Such thinking was certainly justified by the effects of antiviral drugs such as idoxuridine, which is highly toxic to body cells.

Amantadine, developed in the early 1960s, showed few of the exaggerated ill effects of previously developed antivirals but was greeted with extreme suspicion. In fact, if this drug hadn't shown remarkable usefulness in the treatment of a condition completely unrelated to viral infection, its acceptance may well have taken years longer. But under the name Symmetrel, amantadine proved effective against Parkinson's disease. This drug is now widely prescribed as protection against certain strains of type A influenza. It may also lessen the severity of a bout with the flu. Only your doctor can tell you, however, whether amantadine is the wisest disease-fighting strategy in your particular case.

The antibiotic revolution

Penicillin's discovery, in 1938, opened a new era for medicine. For the first time, harmful, invasive bacteria could be destroyed with certainty.

But scientists soon learned that antibiotics in use for a while encourage stronger breeds of bacteria among any that survive an antibiotic dose. The survivors soon reproduce themselves in great numbers, making a new, resistant bacterial strain.

As long as we keep inventing new antibiotics, we stay ahead of the threat— or sometimes we can go back to an earlier antibiotic that has become effective again against a much evolved bacterial strain.

A vaccine is a preparation of killed virus or, sometimes, much-weakened virus that you expose yourself to. When your specialized white blood cells encounter the vaccine, they swing into action just as they would to combat a real infection. Antibodies and memory T cells created in this mock attack will thus be on hand should you make contact with the living, full-strength virus.

Vaccine effects can be dramatic, especially when targeted against a single, identifiable virus. With the aid of vaccines, we have controlled some viral diseases, such as smallpox, measles, and polio. Other vaccines, against more changeable diseases like flu, have greatly reduced the tolls taken in special populations.

Now that you know the nature of cold viruses, you can appreciate the vaccine problem: vaccinate against which of the hundreds of cold viruses? Maybe a few dozen vaccinations, covering the main viral family groups, would give you some immunity, but your protection would be incomplete. Viruses change their shapes from generation to generation, leaving your antibodies waiting to encounter a slightly different form. Additionally, no one knows the identity of the next cold virus, so we can't vaccinate ourselves in advance of it. Why? A vaccine cannot be made up without a purified supply of the virus itself.

Pleurisy

An acute inflammation of the pleura, the delicate membrane that lines the chest cavity and surrounds the lungs, pleurisy is a painful complication of bacterial pneumonia, some viral infections, and other respiratory disorders.

Onset is usually sudden. Chest pain, the main symptom, varies from vague discomfort to (most commonly) an intense stabbing sensation that's most severe when your lungs expand or contract. Depending on the site of pleuritic inflammation, the pain may spread to other areas, such as the shoulder or diaphragm. Fever, dry cough, and difficult breathing, with shallow, rapid respirations, are also common.

Severe pleurisy is often accompanied by or results in pleural effusion—abnormal accumulation of fluid in the pleura and the air spaces of the lungs. If pus is present, you'll have empyema, a severe infection. When pleural effusion or empyema develops, chest pain often subsides.

Treatment of pleurisy consists of pain relief, rest, and antibiotics for infection. For severe pleural effusion, or empyema, the doctor may use a large needle and syringe to remove fluid

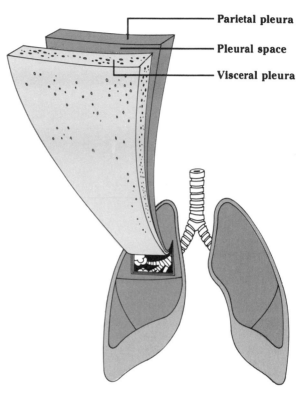

Parietal pleura
Pleural space
Visceral pleura

from between the pleural layers—a procedure known as thoracentesis.

How pleurisy develops

A thin membrane composed of connective tissue, blood and lymph vessels, and smooth muscle fibers, the pleura consist of two layers. The visceral pleura encases the lungs; the parietal pleura lines the inner chest wall. The two layers are normally separated by only a small amount of pleural fluid, which acts as a lubricant when the lungs expand and contract during respiration.

When inflamed, the pleural layers become swollen and congested, hindering normal lubrication by pleural fluid. The resulting friction between the layers during respiration produces the characteristic pain of pleurisy.

Cold complication: Sinus infection

Your sinuses have no sensory nerves to tell you where an infection is located. You'll feel pain, of course, but you may make wrong guesses about its source. Your maxillary sinuses, located below your eyes, are apt to cause sensations like a toothache. Your upper jaw may ache, but so may the upper part of your face or forehead.

Frontal sinuses, located above the eyes, can also become infected, causing pain in the face and forehead.

The ethmoid sinuses are more likely to produce pain behind and between the eyes, sometimes a splitting headache in these areas.

Sphenoid sinuses, located deeper in your facial structure, usually generate a duller ache, difficult to pinpoint. Areas from your forehead and eyes to your temples may be involved.

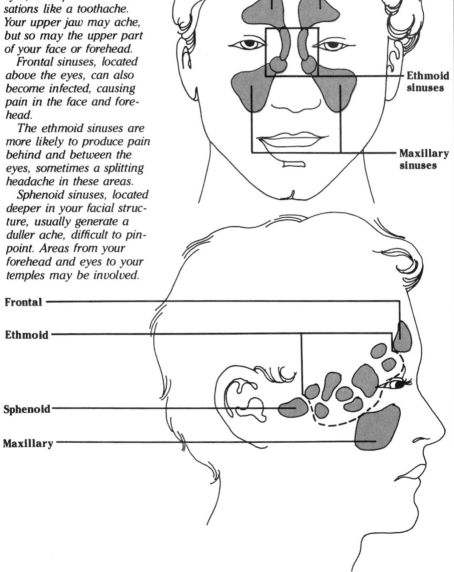

Frontal sinuses

Ethmoid sinuses

Maxillary sinuses

Frontal

Ethmoid

Sphenoid

Maxillary

Cold complication: Ear congestion

If your ear begins to throb, don't blow your nose. Why? The pressure of nose blowing will almost certainly back the congestion up into your eustachian tube. This will interfere with the drainage of mucus and serous fluids from your middle ear. Try drinking warm fluids, such as chicken soup, and perhaps inhaling warm steam. Results won't be dramatic, but you may manage to keep the eustachian tubes open and draining.

If, despite your best efforts, your throbbing and aches increase, you may wish to use a few drops of warm, not hot, mineral oil in the affected ear. However, if signs of infection (fever, chills) persist for more than a half day, or if pain becomes intense, see a doctor immediately. You may need antibiotics to prevent infection complications, such as hearing loss or bone disease within the ear.

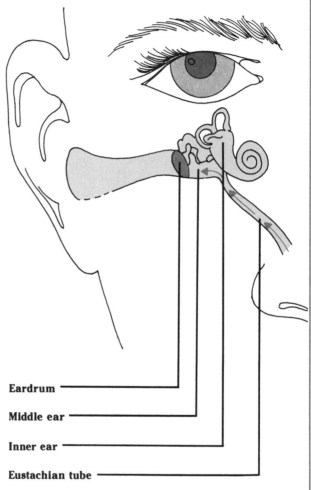

Eardrum

Middle ear

Inner ear

Eustachian tube

Large-scale vaccination against one or more of the chief cold viruses has been tried among volunteers and in the military. Results do show a reduction in colds, but at most a 50% drop in the number of people who catch colds.

Again, a cold isn't a serious disease, and for most of us it doesn't require a vaccination. Slight risks are attached to vaccination, as when the serum brings on allergic reaction or contains active viruses as well as killed or weakened ones. The vaccination risk may

(continued on page 56)

Antibiotics for cold complications

Generic and brand names	Usual adult dosage	Side effects and special considerations
Penicillins		
amoxicillin (Amoxil, Larotid, Polymox, others)	250 to 500 mg by capsule, oral suspension, or chewable tablets every 8 hours	• Watch for signs of penicillin allergy (skin rash, hives, itching, wheezing), nausea, vomiting, and diarrhea and stomach cramps (especially with drugs containing amoxicillin or ampicillin).
amoxicillin/potassium clavulanate (Augmentin)	One 250 or 500 mg tablet every 8 hours (Note: mg strength is based on amount of amoxicillin in the tablet.)	• You should not take any penicillin drugs if you've had an allergic reaction to them. Be sure your doctor, dentist, and pharmacist are aware of your reaction. • Complete your course of treatment, especially if you have a streptococcal infection (strep throat).
ampicillin (Amcill, Omnipen, Polycillin, Principen, others)	250 to 500 mg capsule or oral suspension every 6 hours	• If you miss a dose, take it as soon as you remember it, and space out the next dose by a few hours, if possible. • Drugs containing amoxicillin can be taken with meals. However, all other penicillins should be taken on an empty stomach.
cyclacillin (Cyclapen-W)	250 to 500 mg tablet or oral suspension every 6 hours	• Keep all liquid forms refrigerated. • Check with your doctor or pharmacist before taking any antidiarrhea medicine if diarrhea occurs.
penicillin V (Ledercillin VK, Pen-Vee K, V-Cillin K, others)	125 to 500 mg (200,000 to 800,000 units) tablet or oral solution every 6 to 8 hours	• If you're taking ampicillin or penicillin V, use a contraception method other than birth control pills. • Observe all expiration dates for penicillins.
Cephalosporins		
cefaclor (Ceclor)	250 to 500 mg by capsule or oral suspension every 8 hours	• Watch for skin rash, itching, redness, swelling, nausea, vomiting, and diarrhea. • Complete your course of treatment, especially if you have a streptococcal infection (strep throat).
cefadroxil (Duricef, Ultracef)	500 mg by capsule, tablet, or oral suspension every 12 hours	• Take on either a full or empty stomach. Take with food if stomach distress occurs. • Keep the liquid suspension refrigerated.
cephalexin (Keflex)	250 to 500 mg by capsule, tablet, or oral suspension every 6 hours	• Check with your doctor or pharmacist before taking any antidiarrhea medicine if diarrhea occurs. *(continued)*

Generic and brand names	Usual adult dosage	Side effects and special considerations
Cephalosporins—*continued*		
cephradine (Anspor, Velosef)	250 to 500 mg by capsule or oral suspension every 6 hours	• Urine sugar tests may give false-positive or elevated test results when Clinitest Tablets are used. • Observe all expiration dates for cephalosporins.
Miscellaneous antibiotics		
erythromycin (E-Mycin, ERYC, Erythrocin, Ilosone, others)	250 to 500 mg by capsule, tablet, chewable tablet, or oral suspension every 6 hours	• Watch for diarrhea, nausea, vomiting, upset stomach (cramping and discomfort), yellow eyes or skin, and darkened urine (both may be signs of liver damage). • Complete your course of treatment, especially if you have a streptococcal infection (strep throat). • Be sure you know the proper way to take your drug. Coated tablets and extended-release capsules can't be crushed or chewed. • Check with your pharmacist about whether you should take your medicine on an empty stomach or with meals.
tetracycline (Achromycin V, Sumycin, others)	250 to 500 mg by capsule, tablet, or oral suspension every 6 hours	• Watch for discoloration of infants' or children's teeth, stomach cramps, darkened tongue (from fungal overgrowth), diarrhea, skin sensitivity to light, nausea, and vomiting. • Avoid taking this drug with milk or dairy products. • Take with lots of water to lessen stomach or intestinal upset. • Take with meals if you experience stomach upset. • Stay out of sunlight while you're taking this drug. Wear sunscreen if you must be in the sun.
trimethoprim/ sulfamethoxazole (Bactrim, Septra, others)	1 to 2 tablets or 5 to 10 ml of oral suspension every 12 hours	• Watch for diarrhea, dizziness, headache, appetite loss, nausea, vomiting, itching, or skin rash. • Take on an empty stomach whenever possible. • Drink plenty of liquids while you're taking this drug.

Why your ears pop
*The eustachian tube
(named for a 16th century
Italian anatomist) accounts
for the common sensation
of "popping" ears in air-
planes and elevators where
altitude changes fast. The
tube's whole purpose is to
keep air pressure equal on
both sides of your ear-
drum. Usually air pressure
changes so gradually that
you won't notice any ad-
justments, but a sudden
rise in altitude may cause
a puff of air to escape
quickly from inside your
ear through the eustachian
tube and into your throat.
A sudden inrush of air will
cause the same sensation
when you descend quickly
into denser air.*

be small but then so is the health risk of a cold. Thus, reliable cold vaccination may not only be scientifically impractical; it may not be worth the effort.

Autoimmunity

Your own immune system remains the most effective cold prevention. On the average, people suffer fewer colds as they grow older. This means that antibody stocks grow and diversify, suppressing an ever-wider range of viral types. In other words, you'll slowly immunize yourself against many cold viruses. As far as present medical science goes, you're your best cold protection.

Drugs

Doctors would like to have an immune system back-up—substances that can work in the body to selectively neutralize or destroy viruses. But development of antiviral drugs is only in its infancy. Though a dozen or so antiviral drugs are now in use, they have drawbacks ranging from low effectiveness to dangerous side effects. Still, these antivirals achieve worthwhile results against serious herpes and flu infections.

Because research progresses faster now than a few years ago, thanks to computers and new research technologies (such as recombinant DNA methods), we can look forward to important developments in antiviral drugs.

6

Questions about Catching Colds

We tend to blame colds on any unusual circumstance about ourselves—mood, diet, stress, travel, medical history, for example. The truth, of course, is that no one has perfect immunity to colds, and you most often catch cold through the sheer accident of exposure to one.

Popular notions about how people catch cold aren't always without foundation, though. Science has investigated some commonly held opinions to see how well they hold up against observed groups of cold sufferers. Perhaps your own favorite cold theories are here.

Q: Do people whose tonsils have been removed catch more colds?
A: Apparently not. With or without tonsils, test groups catch about the same number of colds and suffer about equally.

Q: Will wearing wet clothes give you a cold?
A: You may suffer the ill effects of hypothermia (loss of body heat) if you become soaked on a chilly or windy day, which will increase your stress level. Perhaps being chilled won't give you a cold, but the added stress may weaken your defenses.

Q: Do allergies like hay fever make you more vulnerable to colds?
A: Yes, unfortunately, hay fever sufferers catch more colds than the average and often have more severe colds.

Q: Do smokers catch more colds?
A: They don't. But smokers do have worse colds, probably because their respiratory tracts are already chronically irritated by smoking and are more vulnerable to complications.

Q: Is a woman's susceptibility to colds related to her menstrual cycle?
A: Surprisingly, yes, the relationship is strong. Women catch about three times as many colds near the cycle's midpoint than at other times.

Q: **Can you catch cold from someone who already has symptoms?**

A: You certainly can, and you probably will catch a cold if you don't take all the precautions you can think of. Generally, a cold is contagious until your symptoms have clearly begun to fade. At the time your symptoms appear, you actually "shed," or spread, the greatest number of viral particles—through sneezing, coughing, and even conversation.

Q: **Will isolating yourself prevent colds?**

A: Yes, but your isolation must be complete for this technique to work. Studies of populations living on the remotest Scottish islands, where no boats arrive for months at a time, show that colds decline but never quite disappear during isolation. Similar results have turned up among isolated groups of Eskimos and workers in the Antarctic.

Q: **If you already have a viral infection, can you catch another at the same time?**

A: Usually, the first virus to infect a cell takes overall control of the cell's resources—other viruses can't get the cell to "work" for them. Because of this viral interference, you won't have, say, rhinovirus and influenza at the same time. Invading bacteria, however, are in no way hampered by viral activity and often attack in the wake of a virus.

7

Staying Healthy

Physical fitness and colds

Although medical studies continue to look for a relationship between catching colds and physical fitness, no clear-cut answers emerge. Being physically fit has many benefits, but a lower susceptibility to colds isn't one of them. However, fitter people tend to suffer from their cold symptoms about 1 day less than other people.

You can't eliminate colds from your life, but you can reasonably expect fewer colds and usually milder colds when you take sensible health protection measures.

As you now know, your age, sex, and the season are important factors in your likelihood of catching a cold. Strangely, your present health has little to do with it. Ill health doesn't make a cold more likely, only more severe—an added threat to an already weakened body.

Remember, too, that you should avoid strenuous physical activity during any infection, including colds. Respect your body's need for rest. Discontinue your fitness routine until you feel your normal energy returning.

Eating to prevent colds

Your dietary habits may contribute toward preventing colds, but you'll find precise measurements are difficult. Certainly, poor nutrition will make some illnesses more likely, though perhaps not colds. Colds seem to afflict everyone without regard to nutrition. Populations around the world eating an immense variety of foods have generally similar experiences with colds. Still, neglecting your nourishment is a bad idea.

Good nutrition keeps your body's defenses strong. Protein, particularly, is needed to build healthy body tissues, including those in your immune system. A well-balanced diet, including good sources of protein (such as fish, poultry, lean meat, cottage cheese, and yogurt), may not keep you cold-free, but your illnesses will be less miserable.

Vitamin C and colds

In 1970 Linus Pauling, a Nobel Prize–winning chemist, published a book strongly recommending large vitamin C doses to prevent and treat the common cold. Pauling's recommendations have been debated ever since. Dozens of studies, before and after 1970, have failed to resolve the issue. A special problem for researchers studying colds is the sheer number of cold viruses. Perhaps some cold viruses are more sensitive than others to vitamin C's effects. Another,

What about gargles?
*Perhaps advertisements
have told you that antiseptic gargles also improve
your chances of avoiding
colds. They don't. After all,
gargles can only reach a
small area of your throat.
And they don't affect cold
viruses much. The only
gargle of any use to you is
your homemade concoction
to soothe an already irritated throat (see page 84).*

less technical problem for scientists arises from the very personal nature of symptoms. How can we accurately measure and compare cold misery among large numbers of people? Yet, measurements of some kind must be made if we want to know whether a substance such as vitamin C makes a real contribution to relieving suffering.

No one doubts the importance of vitamin C in maintaining healthy body tissues. And vitamin C does seem to contribute to a quick recovery from colds. Pauling suggests, however, that vitamin C can both prevent and *cure* the common cold. The dosage recommended by Pauling for a curative effect (the therapeutic dosage) is quite high, 1 to 2 grams daily or 4 grams and up when you feel a cold coming on. Some people will suffer diarrhea at these dosage levels. If you've decided you want to make your own vitamin C experiment the next time you have a cold, get your doctor's opinion first.

Hygiene

Washing your hands frequently each day works as well as anything else to prevent colds—and more serious illnesses. We all touch our faces without thinking, sometimes bringing viruses or bacteria closer to their preferred invasion routes, the eyes and nose. Washing your hands won't actually kill any infectious agents, but it does remove them from your skin.

Other hygienic measures you may take against colds include: avoiding crowds and people with cold symptoms; keeping your hands away from your eyes and nose; using disposable tissues, not handkerchiefs, to blow your nose, and disposing of them properly; and washing surfaces (such as telephones, light switches, utensils) that are most likely to become contaminated by people with colds.

Fatigue and stress

The role of stress in bringing on a cold has attracted a good deal of scientific attention. Of course, stress can't be exactly measured. Studies do seem to show, though, that sudden changes in your stress level may make you more susceptible to colds. A difficult assignment or new worries that absorb your energies for a few days are the kinds of stress that raise your chances of catching cold. Under such conditions, you might also suffer from lack of sleep. Fatigue may in-

Proper hand washing

When you wash up, you needn't perform a ritual surgical scrub, but do take some care. First, wash your hands several times during the day and always before eating. Use soap and lots of running water. Soap doesn't actually kill many infection sources, but it loosens the oils and deposits on your skin that harbor bacteria and viruses. Running water carries away the contaminants. When you've completed your washing (which may include a good nail scrub),

don't nullify your sensible hygienic practices by drying off on a used towel. In public places, a hot air hand dryer is best, but clean paper towels are certainly acceptable.

If frequent hand washing leaves your hands dry, scratchy, or cracked, use a hand lotion. Use of very strong soaps often causes drying or even allergic skin reactions. You really don't need such soaps to maintain good hygiene.

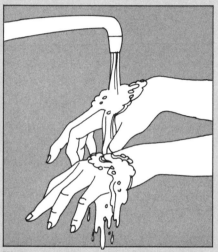

Wet your hands.

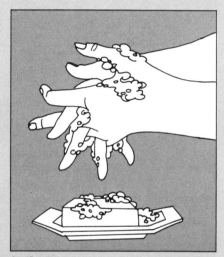

Apply soap.

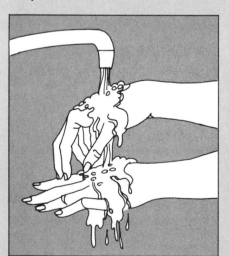

Rinse.

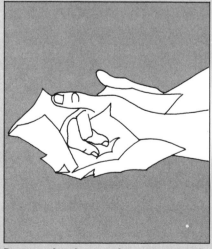

Dry your hands on a clean paper towel.

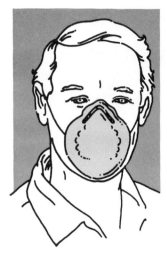

Is a face mask for you?

Disposable paper masks, such as those available in most drugstores, can block the droplets that carry cold viruses. But these masks won't protect you against flu. You'll have to decide for yourself whether wearing a face mask is worth the trouble.

crease your vulnerability.

Reducing stress and getting adequate, restful sleep should be long-term health goals for all of us. Preventing colds is perhaps the very least of the benefits we derive from relaxation and rest.

Can you prevent a cold?

Basic virus research finally yielded, in 1985, a detailed biochemical "map" of the rhinovirus's protein coat. With such a detailed look at the viral exterior, scientists may soon be able to exactly describe the virus's protein receptors, or antigens, that seek out cells in your body. This is perhaps the most important piece of information needed to design the kind of antiviral drug that could neutralize rhinovirus—or other viruses, when their viral maps have also been discovered. The strategy here resembles that of your own immune system's antibodies: design a substance that can plug up a virus's protein tools for gaining entry into healthy cells. Still, such practical and specific cold remedies will take years to develop and test. A little closer to reality is interferon.

Interferon's story is one of great technological success and medical disappointment. To begin with, your immune system produces several natural varieties of interferon, but in the smallest amounts. Interferon hampers viral self-copying after a virus enters a cell. Indeed, interferon showed promise at stopping cancerous growths.

Collecting interferon from human volunteers isn't practical because thousands of pints of human blood yield only an eyedropperful of interferon. Despite interferon's great complexity, it can be manufactured outside the body in useful quantities. The method used, recombinant DNA technology, is at the forefront of current research. Some experts believe that interferon can protect you from rhinovirus—the most common cause of colds. If the new substance passes its FDA tests, you may soon be able to buy an interferon nasal spray to ward off colds.

Antiviral drugs offer a third possibility for preventing colds. Some are available by prescription now. The question with the currently available antiviral drugs isn't so much whether they work against colds but whether they're worth the trouble and expense. Drugs such as amantadine are useful against flu (though not as protective as a vaccine). But are potential side effects like dizziness, insomnia, and anx-

Infection routes

Your digestive and respiratory tracts normally contain a variety of germs (microbes) that give you no trouble. But unwanted viruses and bacteria can be a problem once they gain entry to your body. Once there, they can cause infection. The usual infection routes—through your mouth and nose, eyes, and open sores and fresh wounds—often involve your hands. To control your hands as an infection source, wash them frequently and learn to keep them away from your nose, mouth, and eyes.

Hands. Given the number of things you hold every day, including other human hands, your hands can become your greatest source of potential infection. Wash them frequently during the day.

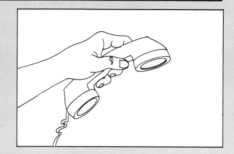

Mouth and nose. Avoid inserting your fingers into your mouth or nose. Try to avoid breathing through your mouth. The likelihood of infection increases with mouth breathing because you dry your protective mucous linings and by-pass the hairlike filtration system in your nose.

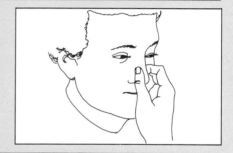

Eyes. Through your eyes' tear (lacrimal) ducts, infection easily finds its way to the nose and so into your respiratory tract. Additionally, your eyes can be sites of painful infections. Usually you bring infection to the eyes by rubbing them with your hands—a habit to avoid.

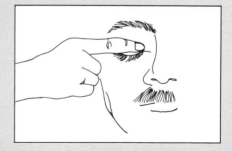

Open sores and fresh wounds. Keep sores and wounds clean and, if possible, covered. Light gauze, which allows air to circulate, stops large airborne particles that may harbor virus and bacteria.

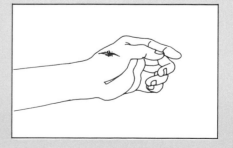

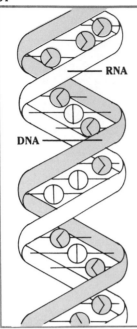

RNA

DNA

Interferon's role

A living cell constantly manufactures the substances it needs for its own growth, repair, and functioning. Plans for everything the cell does are stored inside the nucleus, in long twisted strands of DNA. Carrying out DNA's operating orders is the job of twisted strands of RNA.

Instruction-bearing RNA takes charge of substances, called ribosomes, that float in a cell's interior. Ribosomes follow RNA instructions to manufacture various proteins for use around the cell.

When viral RNA takes over a cell's ribosomes, vital proteins are all diverted into the production of new virus particles. The cell soon dies. If interferon has entered the cell before the virus, it seizes control of the ribosomal machinery, denying the virus an opportunity to subvert the cell's resources.

Remarkably, interferon rarely blocks the use of ribosomes by RNA produced in the nucleus; only the viral RNA is locked out.

iety a reasonable inconvenience for a mild infection like a cold? Besides, amantadine is better at preventing certain viral infections than it is at curing them. You'd have to take such an antiviral drug all year round to keep up your immunity. Another antiviral drug now being tested—and already available in some foreign countries—is ribavirin, sold under the name Virazole. But results aren't available yet to judge if Virazole meets the tests of economy, safety, and effectiveness.

8

The Flu

When flu isn't flu
The "24-hour bug," "stom-ach flu," or "intestinal flu" isn't influenza. Though stomach flu may cause in-testinal symptoms (nausea, vomiting, diarrhea), they're usually not very long-last-ing—seldom more than 2 days. The causes of stom-ach flu haven't been com-pletely identified, and many more are probably as yet undiscovered. One virus thought to be responsible goes by the rather mysteri-ous name Norwalk agent— it was first identified in ill-nesses around Norwalk, Connecticut. Rotavirus, as-trovirus, and others are still being investigated as sources of these fast-hitting intestinal attacks.

Everyone has had a cold, and most people have had, at one time or another, the viruses that cause flu (influenza). Fortunately, the flu viruses are comparatively much fewer than those in the cold-causing groups, and we can trust our immune systems to keep us flu-free for years at a time.

Flu viruses come in three kinds: influenza A, B, or C. Within each group, though chiefly in A, several distinct strains threaten us. Often a newly active strain is named after the geographical location where it was first identified—Hong Kong flu or Singapore flu are examples. A full technical description, however, de-tails the virus's invasion equipment, its antigens.

Influenza viruses carry two kinds of antigen, a neuraminidase that gets the virus past your protec-tive mucous layers, and a hemagglutinin that binds the virus to a target cell, allowing the virus's pirated genetic cargo to spill into a cell's interior. Complete viral names include family (A, B, C), place where first discovered, date discovered, and antigen types (H_1N_1, H_3N_2, and so forth).

Flu epidemics

Unlike colds, flu is apt to infect large numbers of a population at about the same time. It's a disease that can move like a wave across the world from its point of origin. Scientists believe flu's epidemic quality arises from the virus's spectacular ability to alter its own nature.

As we've seen, the number of flu virus types is relatively small. But this is a versatile virus. A flu virus interior contains not a single strand of genetic material, as with most other viruses, but eight sep-arate genetic components. Though you and the rest of the population can develop excellent defenses to a particular virus—virtually closing it down around the world—the flu virus reacts to these defenses by redesigning itself. Actually, the virus is always rede-signing itself, completely accidentally, while it copies itself. How? A flu virus, with its eight complex genetic segments, easily makes mistakes when copying itself. Mistakes that can't work well as viruses—that can't get into a cell, for instance—simply disappear. Some

Kissing and flu

Yes, kissing can spread flu. You should keep in mind, however, that flu is so contagious that just being close enough to kiss will do almost as efficient a job of spreading the virus. Viral particles in large numbers are shed in each breath a flu victim exhales.

bad copies, however, are good viruses and, with a few more generations of workable mistakes, may become so changed as to completely elude antibodies that destroyed their forebears.

Simpler viruses than flu make mistakes, too. Because they're simpler, though, each new generation of, say, rhinovirus will contain fewer, less dramatic mistakes. Your immune system can almost always keep up with the changes in rhinovirus. Your existing antibodies will still recognize a slightly altered rhinovirus, and new, tailored antibodies are soon on the way. Not only does flu outstrip other respiratory viruses, it seems to go into hiding during much of its transformation.

We aren't completely sure where flu viruses hide. We do know that type A infects horses, chickens, and swine as well as humans. The virus spends a few years inside animals performing imperfect self-copying until it finds, once again, that it has become unrecognizable to our immune systems. Whether the flu virus always "drifts" into a new infectious form, changing only a little in each generation, or whether

How flu takes over

When you breathe in a flu virus that attaches to a cell in your respiratory tract, your body reacts. The cell engulfs the virus and tries to destroy it. Chemicals attack the virus cell wall and dis-

solve it, releasing the virus cell contents (primarily genes) into your healthy cell.

The invading genes force your cell to make duplicate genes that arrange themselves into identical bundles. These new viruses—up to 1,000 within 6 hours—burst from your cell and seek out other healthy cells to invade. The invaded cells are destroyed.

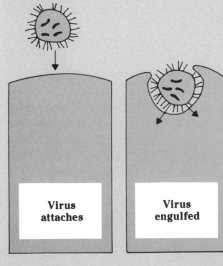
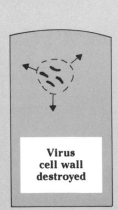
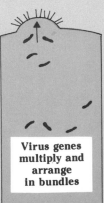

| Virus attaches | Virus engulfed | Virus cell wall destroyed | Virus genes multiply and arrange in bundles |

Can clothes, bed linen, or furniture harbor a flu virus?

Yes, for up to 72 hours. Because the flu virus survives longer outside the body than cold viruses, it may contaminate a variety of surfaces. Even a hardy flu virus, however, can't live indefinitely. You can safely assume that no active viruses are present 2 or 3 days after contamination. In any case, washing contaminated items in hot water destroys the flu virus.

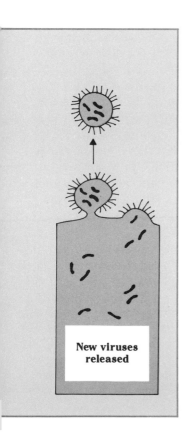

New viruses released

it "shifts" all at once into a radically different form isn't known. Evidence suggests that both kinds of change take place.

Possibly, flu viruses go into cold storage—in the earth's colder regions—where they don't change at all. They have only to wait a few decades to become potent infections once again, when new, unexposed human generations meet them.

A last, troublesome feature of flu virus is its high contagion. Because flu can spread so quickly and easily, epidemics become more probable. Moisture and dust particles so tiny they can drift through the air for hours are vehicles for flu virus. Most cold-carrying particles and droplets fall out of the air within a few minutes. Flu needn't rely much, as colds do, on contact to spread disease.

Whatever the complete answer to flu's epidemic nature, only types A and B are involved. Type C influenza, usually milder than A or B, doesn't spread in an epidemic way; it behaves more like a cold virus. Type A causes most flu illnesses, coming in epidemic waves about every 3 years. Especially widespread and severe disease—a pandemic—occurs perhaps once a decade. Type B is a less frequent visitor, with outbreaks every 5 years or so.

Flu symptoms and treatment

About 2 days after you've been exposed to flu, your symptoms will appear. Flu symptoms strike quickly: you'll know you're sick after only an hour or two. Fever climbs to 102° F. or higher inside a day. Muscle aches and pains are among the first symptoms; cough, sore throat, watery eyes, and headache follow. The worst symptoms should be over within 3 days. Depending on the severity and length of your symptoms, weakness, sweating, and tiredness can last a few days to a few weeks after your viral bout.

Since flu can have serious complications, you shouldn't treat it lightly. Bed rest is essential—and don't try to be too active after your illness, either. Stay in bed while you have symptoms, and don't move around much for a day or two afterwards.

Most of what you should do for flu involves not making your suffering any worse than it has to be. Eat what you want, but don't force food down. Your digestive system isn't up to par while you have flu. Dairy products and raw fruits or vegetables won't go down well. Bland, starchy foods are best—whatever

A century of flu

The four great flu pandemics of the last 100 years are each popularly known by names that suggest a place of origin. The pandemic of 1889 has entered history as the "Asiatic" flu. That most devastating of all flu outbreaks, the 1918 pandemic, is usually called the "Spanish" flu. The more recent visitations of 1957 and 1968 are remembered as the "Asian" and "Hong Kong" flus. All these diseases, of course, were variants of the versatile type A influenza virus.

you find appealing. If you have congestion, use a vaporizer. Gargle for a sore throat. Use cough suppressants for a nonproductive cough. (See page 84 for a simple gargle recipe and advice about cough suppressants.) Don't take painkillers stronger than aspirin or any other medication you may have lying around—drugs your doctor or dentist prescribed for past infections or pain. Inappropriate medications could mask or confuse your symptoms. If you can't keep your fever below 102° F. with aspirin or acetaminophen, see your doctor.

For smokers, having the flu is a good opportunity to quit. The smoke further irritates throat tissues already stripped of protective mucus by your virus.

In short, treat flu as you would treat a cold, but stay in bed longer and watch carefully for complicating symptoms.

The flu pandemic of 1918, the fizzle of 1976

Though not as infamous, perhaps, as the Black Death that swept again and again through the medieval world, disastrous flu outbreaks have regularly visited the world every few decades. Not until deadly flu pandemics of 1889 and 1918 was science really advanced enough to begin asking sensible questions about flu's cause. And not until 1933 did a long trail of dedicated research isolate the flu virus.

In 1918, 500,000 people in the United States died from flu infection. Worldwide, the dead numbered in the millions. We know now the virus responsible for the suffering of 1918 was type A H_1N_1. Our knowledge of it comes chiefly from testing antibodies still circulating in survivors of the pandemic—antibodies can still be detected decades after some illnesses.

This viral strain virtually disappeared by the 1950s only to resurface in 1976. You may remember it as the "swine flu" (swine, too, can host this virus). Naturally, health officials were fearful that a new A H_1N_1 might duplicate the virulence of its 1918 relative. They were able this time to move faster than the virus. Massive doses of vaccine were prepared, 46 million people had shots—and the virus never really arrived. Unpredictable as viral strains are, the type A of 1976 just wasn't the monster of 1918. No one can be sure why; the 1976 strain never exhibited much infectious power, even among groups of people who weren't vaccinated.

Flu complications

Breathing difficulty, coughing up blood, or a bluish color to nails, hands, and face usually mean severe lung infection. See a doctor immediately or get to an emergency room.

Symptoms that don't belong to flu—rash; swollen lymph glands in the neck or groin; swollen, painful joints; whitish pus spots on the back of your throat; or swallowing difficulty—also mean that you'll need a doctor's attention immediately.

A secondary bacterial infection sometimes follows the flu—especially type A flu. If your fever and other symptoms seemed to have peaked but then worsen a day or two later, a secondary infection could be the cause. Or, if your symptoms continue longer than 5 days, you should suspect secondary infection. In either case, consult your doctor as soon as possible.

In children, a grave complication of type B flu (and of measles) is Reye's syndrome. This is a brain infection, an encephalitis, whose cause is unknown. Early signs of possible Reye's syndrome are extreme nausea and vomiting, a high, sustained fever, some loss of memory, and a general sleepiness. Consult a doctor immediately; Reye's syndrome is life threatening (see page 36).

Some research suggests that aspirin taken by children with flu makes Reye's syndrome a little more likely to occur. For this reason, use an aspirin substitute, such as acetaminophen, to control fever whenever you think your child might have flu.

Protecting yourself against flu

You can't do much to prevent flu. Frequent hand washing, staying away from crowds, and avoiding rubbing your eyes and nose help a little, but flu is even more contagious than a cold. Your risk of acute illness and complications is higher if you're over age 60 or pregnant, or have diabetes, or if you suffer from a chronic heart or lung disease—such as emphysema, asthma, or chronic bronchitis. In fact, if you belong to any of these higher risk groups, and a flu outbreak threatens, you should see your doctor about flu vaccination.

Since vaccines take a week or two to build up your antibodies, think about getting flu shots *before* the flu season begins or as soon as possible after a flu outbreak has been reported in your area. (If you're allergic to eggs, be sure to mention it before having a vaccination. Many vaccines are prepared in chicken

Getting over the flu
Bed rest is essential if you have the flu. Don't try to do more than is comfortable until you feel better. In this way, you greatly aid your body's recovery and repair.

eggs.) Even the best vaccine—a vaccine prepared against exactly the right flu strain at exactly the right time—will protect no more than 80% to 90% of recipients.

Some immunity to type A flu virus is achieved with regular doses of amantadine, a prescription drug with proven antiviral qualities. This drug actually blocks contact between flu virus and body cells. Amantadine's protection lasts only as long as you're taking it. Your doctor may prescribe vaccines, or amantadine, or both, depending on your health risks and taking into account what kind of flu virus is going around.

Multipurpose vaccines

When a vaccine immunizes you against one specific viral strain, the vaccine is called monovalent. *A vaccine that acts against two viral strains is termed* bivalent; *against three strains,* trivalent; *and so forth.*

For each new flu season, observers around the globe identify the most active flu strains, and manufacturers prepare that year's vaccine based on these observations. Trivalent vaccines, active against two strains of influenza A and one of influenza B, have been used during the last few years.

9

Allergies

Asthma isn't imagined

Despite popular notions about asthma, this condition isn't an emotional or psychological disorder. Although emotional stress and many other factors (cold air, viral infection, air pollutants, among others) may trigger an asthma attack, they don't cause asthma. Asthma's real cause is a disease, although not well understood, and must be treated medically.

Asthmatics, beware of beta blockers

Some drugs that do exactly the opposite of what bronchodilators do for asthma sufferers are beta blockers. Prescription drugs for the relief of migraine, glaucoma, heart disease, and high blood pressure may contain beta blockers. Asthmatics must strictly avoid any medications that include beta blockers—otherwise, a serious attack may result.

Fortunately, you can easily recognize beta-blocking ingredients because their names all end in -olol (for example, propranolol, pindolol, timolol, nadolol).

When your ever-watchful immune system encounters a substance it doesn't recognize, you're apt to experience a full-scale inflammatory immune response. Even though the "intruder" poses no disease threat, your body may enter the first stages of a disease-fighting reaction. The results are an allergy. Not surprisingly, medical science only began to understand allergies when it could answer basic questions about infection. Both trails, allergies and infections, lead to your body's immune system.

Your immune system is so complex, storing information about so many foreign proteins, that it makes mistakes. But proteins that may provoke an allergic response—in pollens, foods, or animal danders, for example—don't manufacture more of themselves inside your body, as viruses do. Your allergic reaction will only last as long as your immune system needs to dispose of the offending proteins. An allergy attack doesn't last as long, therefore, as a genuine infection. It doesn't take as long to get started, either: noticeable allergy symptoms generally appear within minutes of breathing an allergen (an allergy-producing substance).

Many allergies are triggered by skin contact with an allergen. Such allergies tend to produce skin rashes. An allergen in food might cause you stomach or intestinal upset.

Allergies that cause respiratory symptoms

In your respiratory tract, the principal allergies and symptoms are hay fever and asthma. You'll also want to know about a severe possible allergy complication called anaphylaxis.

Allergies like hay fever, caused by something in the air, can bring on sneezing, nasal congestion, watery eyes, runny nose, and headache. Fever is rare with hay fever, so the name of this ailment is a little misleading. (A medical name for hay fever is allergic rhinitis, or you may prefer another, pollinosis.)

Many effective OTC products are available to treat hay fever. Most contain an antihistamine, which counteracts the inflammatory alarm spread by the hista-

What happens in asthma

Here's what happens when a person with asthma inhales an allergen.

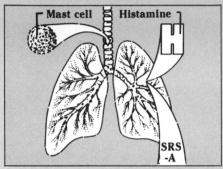

1. In response to an allergen, IgE antibodies are produced. These antibodies trigger the breakdown of mast cells in the lung tissue and the release of histamine and the slow-reacting substance of anaphylaxis (SRS-A).

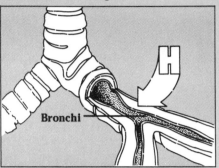

2. Release of histamine in the large airways (bronchi) causes bronchial irritation, redness, and swelling (inflammation).

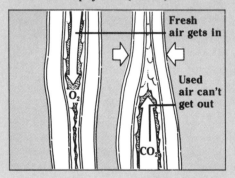

5. When the person inhales, the airway can still enlarge enough to allow air to reach the lung's gas exchange units (alveoli). However, when the person tries to exhale, the swollen lung airways block the air's exit. Air gets into the alveoli—but can't get out.

mine produced in mast cells. Antihistamines also have the welcome effect of helping to dry mucus in your congested air passages and sinuses.

Another class of drug useful to hay fever sufferers is decongestants. These shrink swollen membranes. They can help relieve sinus pressure and stuffiness, something that antihistamines don't do quickly. Many allergy relief products contain both an antihistamine and a decongestant.

Read the label

Read the label on any allergy medication you decide to try. Frequently, the label warns of drowsiness caused by antihistamines. You might not wish to drive or work around potentially dangerous equipment after taking an antihistamine. Never exceed the label's recommended dosage limits. Nose sprays, nose drops,

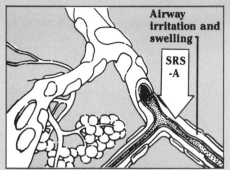

3. Release of SRS-A causes swelling of the small airways and attracts a hormonelike substance called prostaglandin, which works with histamine.

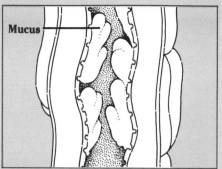

4. Prostaglandins and histamines increase mucus production, which further narrows the airways.

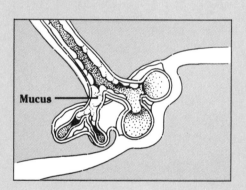

6. As mucus fills the airways and alveoli, normal air exchange can't take place.

or inhalants will probably contain decongestants. Use them sparingly—dosing yourself with decongestants for more than a few days will lead eventually to greater congestion, not less. Oral decongestants, those taken by mouth in pill or liquid form, can cause a racing heartbeat or a blood pressure increase. Avoid taking oral decongestants if you have high blood pressure or hyperthyroidism or take MAO inhibitors for depression.

Because an allergy sufferer has no underlying infection, he won't need an antibiotic. Antibiotics themselves can cause allergic reactions and so may actually contribute to an allergy crisis.

Asthma

Sudden wheezing, coughing, tightness in the chest, and shortness of breath could signal an asthma at-

(continued on page 76)

Desensitizing your home

If yours is a troublesome allergy, you'll benefit from ridding your home as far as possible of offending allergens. Hay fever sufferers, for example, benefit greatly from filtered indoor air. Anyone sensitive to airborne allergens (pollen, dust, fungal spores) should change air-conditioning or heating system filters frequently. Frequent housecleaning often helps, too. A dry, dust-free basement is particularly important.

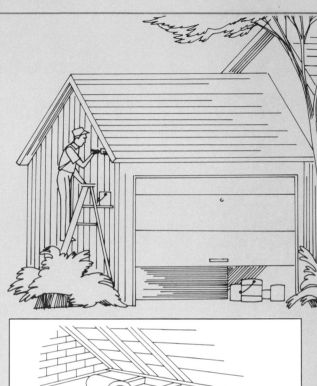

Household dust sources may be too numerous to eliminate completely, but check these sources: bare bricks and wood; old, chalky paint; exposed insulation; deteriorating fabrics and carpets; and poorly filtered air heating and cooling systems. Wood and brick surfaces can be sealed, old paint scraped away, insulation covered, and filters changed regularly.

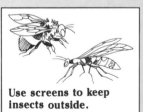

Cover insulation.

Here are representative protective actions you can take in your home:

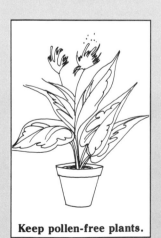

Keep pollen-free plants.

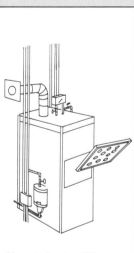
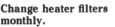

Change heater filters monthly.

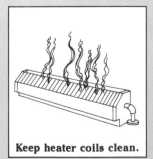

Use screens to keep insects outside.

Keep heater coils clean.

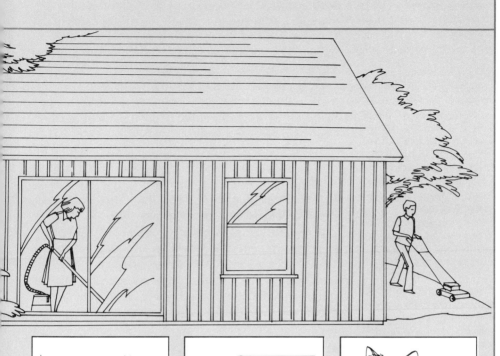

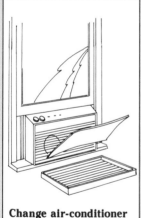

Change air-conditioner filters monthly.

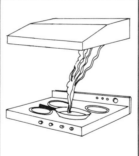

Use a kitchen exhaust fan.

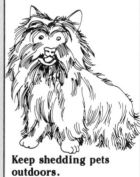

Keep shedding pets outdoors.

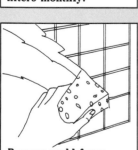

Remove mold from bathrooms.

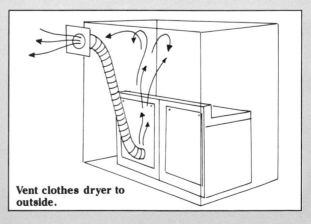

Vent clothes dryer to outside.

Asthma drugs

Though some bronchodilators are available over the counter, you shouldn't use them without a doctor's advice. Bronchodilators, remember, are potent medicines sold for the relief of a very specific and common complaint: asthma. Overdoses of these medications or simultaneous use with drugs like beta blockers (propranolol [Inderal]) or antidepressants can cause serious side effects.

Most bronchodilators simulate to some extent the effects of adrenaline. Active ingredients include albuterol (salbutamol), ephedrine, epinephrine, isoetharine mesylate, isoproterenol, metaproterenol, terbutaline, or theophylline and its derivatives (aminophylline, dyphylline, and oxtriphylline).

Brand-name medications prepared with these ingredients for use as bronchodilators include Alupent, Bronkosol, Isuprel, Metaprel, Primatene, Proventil, and Ventolin. Another kind of asthma medication, cromolyn sodium, (Intal, Nasalcrom) isn't a bronchodilator and won't help an asthma attack—it's used strictly to prevent asthma attacks. Beclomethasone (Vancenase, Vanceril) is another asthma preventive. Neither should be used during an attack.

tack. Asthma symptoms happen when branching airways inside the lungs suddenly narrow. Spasms in the muscle sheaths surrounding the airways are the cause. Very sticky mucus soon forms in the airways, further restricting the airflow.

Although asthma can be an allergic symptom, infection, stress, smoking, fumes, or just cold air can bring on an attack. See your doctor about treating your asthma and finding its cause.

If you know you have asthma, you've probably already discussed it with your doctor. With medical advice, you know when and how to use bronchodilators, drugs that ease bronchial muscle spasms. Bronchodilators are available over the counter. The FDA says that several ingredients are effective: ephedrine, epinephrine, theophylline, and methoxyphenamine hydrochloride. But these drugs are only for temporary relief. If your asthma doesn't ease after 20 minutes to an hour, or you can't catch your breath at all, call your doctor or have someone take you to an emergency room.

Repeated use or overdose of bronchodilators can raise your heart rate and blood pressure, and cause nervousness, nausea, or vomiting. These are powerful drugs.

What are you allergic to?

If your allergy seems to occur only at certain times of year, you probably have hay fever. Sneezing attacks in the spring usually signal an allergy to tree pollens. Almost any leafy tree, or several of them, could be responsible. Summer attacks are more likely due to grass or weed pollens. In the fall, weed pollens alone cause most hay fever. Sensitivity to many kinds of pollen can lengthen the hay fever season for some sufferers, making life miserable for months at a time. Winter symptoms may result from molds, dust, or dust mites.

When hay fever symptoms appear at irregular times and seasons over the course of a few years, pollens probably aren't the culprits. Feathers, house dust, animal dander, and funguses may also cause allergic rhinitis—the same thing as hay fever, but specialists usually reserve the term *hay fever* just for pollen allergies.

Often, you'll know exactly what to avoid. If you sneeze only when you're around cats, the obvious

(continued on page 80)

How to use a bronchodilator

Inhaling the medication in a bronchodilator will help an asthmatic person breathe more easily. Here's how to use a bronchodilator.

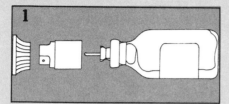

Remove the mouthpiece and cap from the bottle. Then remove the cap from the mouthpiece.

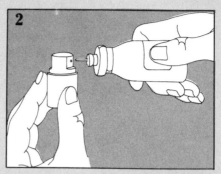

Turn the mouthpiece sideways. On one side of the flattened tip, you'll see a small hole. Fit the metal stem on the bottle into the hole.

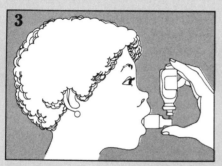

Now exhale. Hold the bronchodilator upside down, as shown here, and close your lips loosely around the mouthpiece.

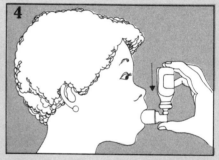

Inhale slowly. As you do, firmly push the bottle against the mouthpiece—one time only—to release one dose of medicine. Continue inhaling until your lungs feel full.

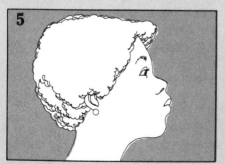

Take the mouthpiece away from your mouth, and hold your breath momentarily.

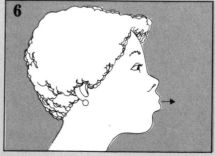

Purse your lips and exhale slowly. If the doctor suggests, repeat the procedure. Finally, rinse the mouthpiece with warm water. Important: Never overuse your bronchodilator. Follow your doctor's instructions exactly.

Antihistamines

Antihistamines can help control your runny nose and sneezing, but they cause side effects like drowsiness that you'll have to consider.

Drug	Usual adult dosage	Special considerations
azatadine maleate (Optimine)	1 to 2 mg every 8 to 12 hours as needed	
brompheniramine maleate (Dimetane, Dimetapp Extentabs)	4 mg every 4 to 6 hours, as needed; for extended-release tablets, 8 to 12 mg every 8 to hours, as needed	• Sedative effects are less pronounced. • Also available as an elixir
carbinoxamine maleate (Clistin)	4 to 8 mg every 6 to 8 hours, as needed	• Sedative effects are more pronounced.
chlorpheniramine maleate (Chlor-Trimeton, Teldrin, Chlor-Trimeton Repetabs)	4 mg every 4 to 6 hours, as needed; for extended-release capsules, 8 to 12 mg every 8 to 12 hours, as needed	• Sedative effects are less pronounced. • Also available as a syrup
clemastine fumarate (Tavist)	1.34 mg two times daily or 2.68 mg one to three times daily, as needed	• Sedative effects are less pronounced.
cyproheptadine hydrochloride (Periactin)	4 mg every 6 to 8 hours, as needed	• May cause increased appetite • Also available as a syrup

General advice

• Call your doctor if you experience the following while taking antihistamines:
—sore throat
—fever
—unusual bleeding or bruising
—unusual tiredness or weakness.
• For all antihistamines except terfenadine, sedation and drowsiness occur frequently. Don't attempt to drive a car or operate heavy machinery until you've become accustomed to, and are able to safely predict, how the antihistamine affects you.
• Other less common side effects are:
—thickening of bronchial secretions
—blurred vision or any change in vision
—confusion
—difficult or painful urination
—dizziness
—dryness of mouth, nose, or throat
—increased skin sensitivity to sun
—appetite loss (increased appetite with cyproheptadine)
—nightmares
—ringing or buzzing sound in ears
—skin rash
—stomach upset or stomach pain (more common with tripelennamine)
—unusual excitement, nervousness, restlessness, or irritability
—unusual increase in sweating
—unusually fast heartbeat.
• Children and elderly patients are usually more sensitive to the effects of

Drug	Usual adult dosage	Special considerations
dexchlorpheniramine maleate (Polaramine, Polaramine Repetabs)	2 mg every 6 to 8 hours, as needed; extended-release tablets, 4 to 6 mg every 8 to 12 hours, as needed	• Sedative effects are less pronounced. • Also available as a syrup
diphenhydramine hydrochloride (Benadryl)	25 to 50 mg every 4 to 6 hours, as needed	• Sedative effects are more pronounced. • Also available as a syrup and as an elixir
diphenylpyraline hydrochloride (Hispril)	5 mg every 12 hours, as needed	
phenindamine tartrate (Nolahist)	25 mg every 4 to 6 hours, as needed	
terfenadine (Seldane)	60 mg every 8 to 12 hours, as needed	• Sedative effects not likely to occur.
tripelennamine hydrochloride (PBZ, PBZ-SR)	25 to 50 mg every 4 to 6 hours, as needed; extended-release tablets, 100 mg every 8 to 12 hours as needed	• May upset your stomach • Also available as an elixir
triprolidine hydrochloride (Actidil)	2.5 mg every 6 to 8 hours, as needed	• Sedative effects are less pronounced. • Also available as a syrup

antihistamines. Confusion, difficult and painful urination, dizziness, drowsiness, feeling faint, or dryness of mouth, nose, or throat may be more likely to occur in elderly patients. Also, nightmares or unusual excitement, nervousness, restlessness, or irritability may be more likely to occur in children and in elderly patients.

• If you take antihistamines regularly, make sure your doctor knows if you're taking large amounts of aspirin (for, say, arthritis or rheumatism). Effects of too much aspirin, such as ringing in the ears, may be covered up by the antihistamine.

• Antihistamines will add to the effects of alcohol and other central nervous system (CNS) depressants (medicines that slow down the nervous system, possibly causing drowsiness). Some examples of CNS depressants are sedatives, tranquilizers, or sleeping medicine; prescription pain medicine or narcotics; barbiturates; medicine for seizures; muscle relaxants; or anesthetics, including some dental anesthetics. Check with your doctor before taking any of the above while you are using an antihistamine.

• Take the drug with food or a glass of water to lessen stomach irritation, if necessary.

• If you're taking the extended-release tablet form, swallow the tablets whole. Don't break, crush, or chew them.

How hay fever got its name

Long before allergies were ascribed to the complex workings of your immune system, people associated such attacks with outdoor activities in the summer and fall. Getting in the year's several hay crops was special misery for certain people. Naturally, some people concluded that newly cut hay must somehow be responsible.

Many kinds of hay do belong to the family of grasses whose pollen causes allergic reactions. We may refer to hay fever a little more accurately today as pollinosis, naming the real culprit, but the hay fever name has stuck, whether your allergy is actually caused by tree pollens, weed pollens, or genuine grass pollens.

Allergy culprits

Though a list of everything that causes an allergy would run to many pages, here are the kinds of substances that cause the overwhelming majority of allergy misery:

• pollens
• dust
• dust mites
• powders (including cosmetics)
• animal dander
• mold spores
• hair particles
• fabric particles
• seeds
• flour
• beef
• insect dust (feces)
• feathers
• fumes (paint, insecticide, exhaust)
• perfumes
• tobacco smoke.

conclusion is an allergy to cat dander. But, the cause of your particular allergy may elude you. Your detective work will be especially difficult if you happen to have multiple allergies, making a trial-and-error approach too complicated.

Medical tests can uncover the causes of most allergies. A common test employs carefully spaced rows of scratches on the skin. A different possible irritant, or allergen, is injected between the skin layers. Those scratches that become reddened or swollen indicate troublesome substances. With this knowledge, you'll be better able to avoid the chief irritants to your immune system. You could also prepare yourself before any likely exposure by taking a small antihistamine dose. Consult your doctor about appropriate drugs and doses.

For allergy sufferers who can't get away from their allergies (house dust, for instance), a doctor may attempt desensitization. Starting with minute amounts and progressing slowly to larger quantities, he'll inject you with the allergen. Over time—it may take years—the immune system seems to lose interest in the allergen. Desensitization means a long treatment, expense, and a small risk of exaggerated, severe allergic symptoms during the treatment. Still, it's worth the trouble when nothing else can relieve constant allergy misery.

Desensitization probably speeds up a process that takes place naturally in most people with allergies. Most sufferers find that hay fever and other allergies tend to diminish with age. But you can't predict with certainty whether or not you'll suffer in a new hay fever season.

10 Coughs

Don't make your cough worse

Since antihistamines have the effect of drying up the secretions in your respiratory tract, don't use them when you have a cough—you don't want to dry your mucus secretions and make your cough less productive.

Coughing is a healthy, necessary reflex to expel foreign objects or excess fluids from your airway. You must keep in mind, when you decide to treat a cough, that your cough may be helping your body cope with infection.

A *productive* cough—one that brings mucus up through your throat—clears your airway. A *nonproductive* cough—dry, hacking, painful—more likely is triggered by dry, inflamed tissue in your throat. All your respiratory surfaces are coated normally with mucus. The tissue underneath mucous layers becomes irritated when exposed to the continuous air currents of your breathing. You might have experienced this as a ticklish throat. Some respiratory viruses can dissolve mucus (in order to attack tissue underneath). Other viruses migrate down the hairlike cilia to reach their targets. Either way, you'll have a cough and a dry, painful throat.

As long as your cough is doing what it's supposed to—moving mucus out of your respiratory tract—don't try to stop it. When your cough is no longer productive, you may want relief for a sore throat and dry, nagging cough. Such coughs are usually the result of infection, but not necessarily. Hot, very dry air can dry up the mucous secretions in your throat and lead to a persistent ticklish cough. You may need to do nothing more than moisten your throat (or moisturize the air around you) to stop this cough. For coughs with infection, you'll want to take other measures.

Why you cough

Different kinds of cough medication and treatment are aimed at different parts of the coughing process. Here's that process:

A cough begins when detector nerve endings in your respiratory tract become irritated enough to send cough signals to the brain. These signals could mean obstruction in an airway, or the presence of chemical or infectious irritants. Some cough signals can actually originate elsewhere: from the diaphragm, from the protective sac around your lungs (the pleura), and even from the ear.

Types of coughs

Coughs come, basically, in two kinds: productive coughs, which bring up sputum; and nonproductive coughs, which are dry and scratchy. Don't try to interfere with a productive cough. You can make the cough more productive still by drinking warm fluids or inhaling warm steam. Let a productive cough do its job clearing mucus from your respiratory tract. Treat a nonproductive cough with soothing syrups, lozenges, or suppressants, if you wish.

See your doctor about chronic coughing, any cough that doesn't seem to go away, and coughing that brings up col-ored (yellow, greenish, brown, or pink) or foul-smelling sputum.

A few special coughs often indicate a particular disease or condition: Coughing in bursts followed by a "whooping" intake of breath suggests whooping cough (pertussis). Hoarse, barking coughs usually accompany croup. And sudden wheezing, coughing attacks with shortness of breath may be caused by asthma.

Sharp pain on coughing isn't normal and can mean a fractured rib. See your doctor about any coughing symptom you think out of the ordinary.

All cough signals converge in the lowest part of the brain, called the medulla. Information passes from the medulla to higher parts of your brain—and you become aware that you need to cough. If the signal isn't very strong, you can ignore it. Stronger signals are more urgent, as for example when you've inhaled a little bit of water that you intended to swallow.

When your brain says cough, the decision is relayed again through the medulla and sent to your epiglottis and breathing muscles, the diaphragm. The epiglottis quickly closes down over your windpipe, blocking it. At the same time your diaphragm contracts, causing air pressure to build in the lungs. When the epiglottis suddenly opens, it releases a pressurized rush of air that carries your airway obstructions or irritants upward.

Two cough suppressants

To suppress a cough, then, you'll need either to soothe the nerves that send signals or calm the brain's cough center, where the decision to cough is made. Both theories are at work in cough suppressants you may buy over the counter.

Cough suppressants acting on irritated nerve endings include two types: local anesthetics and demulcents. Local anesthetics can soothe a raw throat but not, says the FDA, in the small doses contained in OTC products. Leave the prescription of local anesthetics to your doctor. Demulcents help to form soothing, protective coatings in your throat, reducing irritation. You'll recognize them as cough syrups and throat lozenges. A demulcent's ingredients might include honey, licorice, glycerin, acacia, wild cherry, camphor, menthol, and eucalyptus oil. All are safe, according to the FDA, but not necessarily effective. Remember, too, that many syrups contain alcohol, sometimes as much as you would find in wine. Diabetics may wish to avoid using alcoholic or sugary medications. Alcohol can multiply the effects of other drugs, such as sedatives, antidepressants, and tranquilizers. You shouldn't take any alcohol while using these medications.

Active ingredients

Cough suppressants that work on the cough center will probably contain one of three active ingredients found safe and effective by the FDA: codeine, dextromethorphan, or diphenhydramine hydrochloride. Codeine is derived from opium and can be habit-forming; it's not available in OTC products in many states. Codeine isn't considered at all dangerous for the occasional treatment of coughs—that's something codeine does better than almost any other drug. Dextromethorphan runs a close second to codeine's effectiveness, is non–habit-forming, and is free of side effects when used as indicated on labels. None of these cough remedies should be given to children under 2.

Another kind of cough medicine, called an expectorant, thins the secretions that cause congestion, so coughing can bring them up. But the FDA says no OTC expectorant does an effective job. Drinking warm fluids and inhaling steam are far more effective expectorants and are very inexpensive.

Antihistamines and decongestants have no effect on coughs. Don't use them; they might actually complicate the symptoms of your cough.

For special kinds of coughs, with asthma, for example, you may need special drugs. Bronchodilators, for asthma, can be purchased over the counter; that doesn't mean bronchodilators are safe. You should follow your doctor's advice in using any bronchodilator, whether by prescription or over the counter. *Never* use a bronchodilator in the hopes of clearing up congestion. These are powerful drugs, capable of relaxing breathing muscles, but they do nothing at all for colds or flu, unless complicated by asthma.

Recipe for a cough gargle
1 cup warm water
1 teaspoon salt
Dissolve the salt in the warm water. You can mix more if you wish, but maintain about the same proportion of salt to water. (Don't drink this mixture; it's only for gargling to soothe an inflamed throat.)

Bronchodilators can have serious side effects, which include a racing heartbeat and elevated blood pressure.

No doubt you can find something in your drugstore that will relieve a cough. Over 800 products for cough are on shelves around the country. You're familiar now with ingredients that work. As the FDA has pointed out, the product with the most ingredients isn't necessarily the best. According to government tests, OTC products often contain ingredients in amounts too small to work effectively. Local anesthetics and antibacterial agents usually belong to this category.

Some products combine ingredients in an illogical way. Adding an expectorant to an antihistamine makes no sense because one drug tries to produce more fluids while the other acts to dry them. Far more sensible is the combination of a suppressant with a demulcent, soothing the cough center and irritated tissue at the same time. No OTC medication, however, can do better than to ease your cough. Your cough won't disappear because of cough medicine.

Treating a cough without drugs

What you can or should accomplish with OTC drugs is limited. The most important thing you can do for a tight, productive cough is to drink warm liquids and inhale warm, *not hot,* steam. Adding other ingredients to steam, like eucalyptus oil, has no detectable extra cough benefit, though they may make your sickroom more pleasantly fragrant.

You can make your own demulcents for a cough that has become dry and nonproductive. Moisture is still the most important part of treatment. Adding honey to tea or hot milk may relieve a dry, irritated throat. Sucking on a piece of hard candy works quite well, too. Or you might try a gargle of 1 cup of warm water with 1 teaspoon of salt. If you smoke, give it up at least for the duration of your cough. Smoking worsens throat irritation and throat and lung cell damage.

If nothing works, if your cough lasts a week or more, or if you have any symptoms of complications, see your doctor.

Cough complications

Symptoms that are out of the ordinary for coughs don't automatically mean you have a serious disease,

Why and how you cough

Coughing is your body's way of removing irritants and obstructions from your airway. It's a four-stage process: (1) sensory nerves detect an irritant or obstruction; (2) the sensory signals travel to your brain (the medulla); there, the decision to cough or not to cough is made; (3) a cough decision is relayed to muscles in your epiglottis to seal off lungs and to muscles between your ribs and diaphragm; air pressure within your lungs rises; (4) the epiglottis opens, releasing a pressurized burst of air that propels the irritant or obstruction upward and out of your airway. All of this can happen so quickly that you weren't even aware you were about to cough.

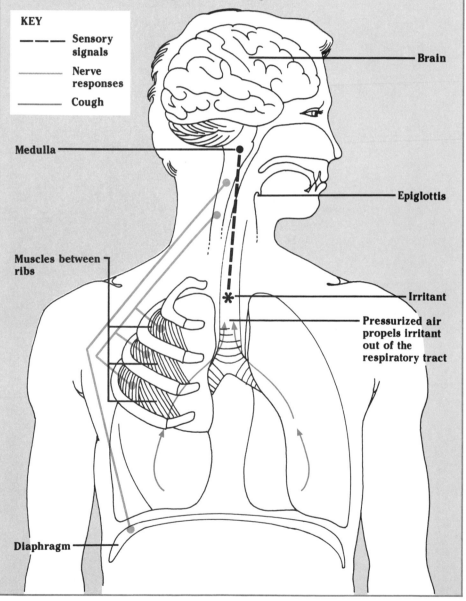

KEY
- – – – Sensory signals
- ——— Nerve responses
- ——— Cough

Brain

Medulla

Epiglottis

Muscles between ribs

Irritant

Pressurized air propels irritant out of the respiratory tract

Diaphragm

Broken ribs

Believe it or not, broken ribs can occur as a complication of cold or flu. How? Severe coughing can put excessive stress on the inner chest wall—possibly enough stress to break a rib. This rarely occurs in young, otherwise healthy persons, but it's a real and potentially serious problem in elderly persons, especially those suffering from osteoporosis—a metabolic disorder that causes the bones to become brittle and abnormally susceptible to fractures. A broken rib is not only excruciatingly painful; it can also cause serious com-plications, among them a punctured lung or lacerated blood vessels.

So if you feel a sudden, unusually sharp and severe chest pain, accompanied by tenderness and swelling over the affected area, you may have broken a rib. You may even be able to feel the break or fracture.

What should you do? Get yourself to a doctor immediately for a chest X-ray. Don't wrap your chest with bandages; this only restricts normal chest movement and could cause further complications.

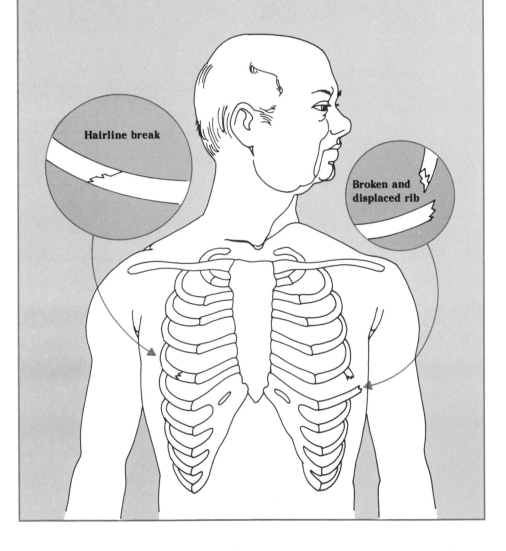

Hairline break

Broken and displaced rib

but you should see a doctor. You must see a doctor or visit an emergency room if you develop any of these complications:

Three serious cough complications

Breathing difficulty. *Shortness of breath or wheezing can happen when your lungs are congested or when airways inside the lung contract in size. Another sign to watch for is a bluish color to fingernails or face.*
Painful breathing. *This could mean a fractured bone. Powerful or constant coughing can fracture ribs, especially in older people, who often suffer calcium loss from bones. Any spot on your rib-* *cage that remains painful to the touch could be a fracture. Painful breathing might also indicate infection of the protective sacs that surround the lungs (pleurisy) and heart (pericarditis).*
Coughing blood. *Blood isn't always obvious when mixed with mucus. Reddish, rust-colored, or brown mucus might contain blood. Usually, you'll see any blood that is present as more obvious, bloody streaks in sputum.*

Disease and coughing

Some diseases cause coughs that help identify a particular infection. You should be able to recognize these coughs. Most coughs, however, aren't so distinctive; they merely mean that any one of several hundred viruses has infected your respiratory tract.

Fever and spasmodic coughing—rapid uncontrollable bursts of coughing—followed by gasps for breath accompany whooping cough (pertussis). The "whoop" comes after a fit of coughing; the first deep gasp often makes a high-pitched sound as it travels down a congested airway. Children are most likely to have this disease. Though whooping cough is often no more than a nuisance, this bacterial infection can be quite serious in the young child, particularly those under age 2.

A loud barking, honking cough occurs with croup, a complication of simple colds, usually in children. Unusual amounts of mucus are produced in the lower throat. This makes breathing noisy and a little labored. A child may become terrified at the choking, stifling sensation, but the remedy is quick and easy. Have your child inhale steam from a bathroom shower or basin of hot water. If steam doesn't ease your child's breathing within 20 minutes or so, call your doctor or take the child to an emergency room.

A chronic cough accompanied by wheezing may indicate either emphysema or chronic bronchitis. Both afflictions can contribute to an equally serious, similar problem referred to as COPD (chronic obstructive

The tenacity of whooping cough
Whooping cough, a bacterial disease, can last a long time—6 weeks or more. Its first stage resembles a cold; the distinctive cough doesn't begin until stage two, a week or so after coldlike symptoms appear. The third, or convalescent, stage ushers in an easing of symptoms, but occasional coughing fits may happen for weeks.

Smokers' cough?

Cough that happens mostly when you get up every morning probably means you're a smoker—you'd better think about giving up the habit soon. Chronic morning cough might also be an early sign of tuberculosis, particularly if you produce yellow or blood-streaked sputum. See a doctor for testing.

pulmonary disease). And both take years to develop. The symptoms worsen so slowly and subtly that you may try to ignore them. See a doctor as soon as you identify your symptoms.

Sudden coughing attacks, wheezing, and shortness of breath could be asthma. Asthma attacks can last from minutes to hours, even days. Your doctor will help determine the cause. Many drugs are available to relieve asthma symptoms, but all should be used only with a doctor's instructions.

These aren't the only diseases that cause cough—just a few with unusual coughs. Flu, cold, measles, and pneumonia often bring coughs. Your other symptoms—fever, runny nose, rash, swelling, breathing difficulty—will persuade you whether to see your doctor or to rest at home and try to endure. Look and listen for anything unusual about your cough. Coughing up yellow or greenish sputum, or foul-smelling sputum, might mean a lung infection you're not even aware of. Coughs that last more than a week, even without other symptoms, should be checked by a doctor. Your cough might be caused by an irritant at your workplace or home, or it could signal changes in your respiratory tract, growths such as polyps or tumors. Whatever the cause, you'll want to identify it as soon as possible.

Staying healthy vs. smoking

No discussion of respiratory illnesses can be complete without a few words about smoking. By now, no one in America would argue that smoking is an unhealthy habit. The surgeon general's report on smoking's adverse effects has grown to over a thousand pages of bad news for smokers. As far as colds and coughs are concerned, the bad news is usually chronic bronchitis. Since smoking causes most chronic bronchitis, it causes most of the chronic coughs in this country.

Smokers tend to ignore the beginnings of ill health. The characteristic morning cough—smoker's cough—may be overlooked. Smokers come to believe this cough is just a normal part of getting up each morning. It's not, of course; it's symptomatic of chronic bronchitis. For these and many other reasons, smokers should persuade themselves to quit.

Quitting smoking

Unfortunately, quitting is tough because nicotine is addictive. Only about one out of every five smokers

(continued on page 92)

Nonprescription Cough Medications

If you want to avoid certain cough medicine ingredients like antihistamines or alcohol, this chart can guide you.

Product	Cough suppressant	Expectorant	Decongestant	Antihistamine	Alcohol
Benylin DM	dextromethorphan	—	—	—	Yes
Cheracol Plus	dextromethorphan	—	phenylpropanolamine	chlorpheniramine	Yes
Codimal DM	dextromethorphan	—	phenylephrine	pyrilamine	Yes
Comtrex liquid	dextromethorphan	—	phenylpropanolamine	chlorpheniramine	Yes
Delsym	dextromethorphan	—	—	—	No
Fedahist Expectorant	—	guaifenesin	pseudoephedrine	chlorpheniramine	No
Formula 44 Cough Mixture	dextromethorphan	—	—	doxylamine	Yes
Head & Chest	—	guaifenesin	phenylpropanolamine	—	Yes
Lanatuss Expectorant	—	guaifenesin, sodium citrate, and citric acid	phenylpropanolamine	chlorpheniramine	No
Novahistine Cough & Cold Forumla	dextromethorphan	—	pseudoephedrine	chlorpheniramine	Yes
NyQuil (Nighttime)	dextromethorphan	—	pseudoephedrine	doxylamine	Yes
Pertussin 8 Hour	dextromethorphan	—	—	—	Yes
Robitussin-PE	—	guaifenesin	pseudoephedrine	—	Yes
Romilar CF	dextromethorphan	—	—	—	Yes
Romilar III	dextromethorphan	—	phenylpropanolamine	—	Yes
Triaminic Expectorant	—	guaifenesin	phenylpropanolamine	—	Yes

Tuberculosis

An acute or chronic infection caused by various strains of mycobacteria, tuberculosis (TB) continues to affect many people. Although worldwide incidence dropped dramatically in the mid-20th century, it may now actually be increasing. Why? Among other factors, increased use of drugs that suppress the body's immune system and increased opportunities for travel are exposing more and more people to the mycobacterium bacteria, for which they may have little or no immunity. Incidence still is highest in undeveloped countries, where people are more apt to live in crowded, poorly ventilated conditions. But although TB is less common in the United States, in certain areas with a large population of recent immigrants, incidence has risen to the same levels as in the immigrants' countries of origin.

TB is a particularly difficult disease to prevent, because it's typically so unpredictable. After exposure to TB, only about 5% of persons develop an active infection within a year. In the remainder, microorganisms cause an infection that produces no symptoms. The body's immune system usually controls the bacteria by killing it or by walling it up inside a tiny nodule known as a tubercle. Then, the bacteria may lie dormant for many years, only to reactivate and spread at any time, causing active infection. Tubercles usually develop in the lungs, but may also spread to other parts of the body, such as the lymph nodes and kidneys. Certain factors increase the likelihood of reactivation of infection, among them uncontrolled diabetes, alcoholism, leukemia, Hodgkin's disease, and treatment with corticosteroids or immunosuppressive drugs.

Exposure to TB usually results from an infected person's cough or sneeze. Inhaling airborne particles may introduce bacteria into the lungs. They then travel through the lymphatic system, to

TUBERCLE

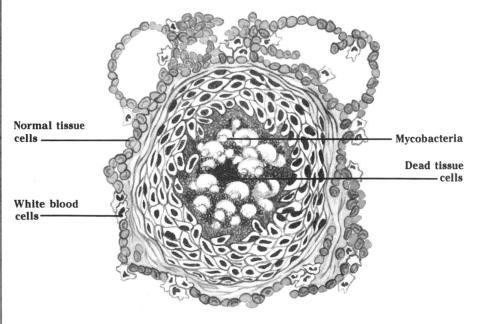

Normal tissue cells

White blood cells

Mycobacteria

Dead tissue cells

Arrows on this X-ray of a person with TB indicate location of tubercles.

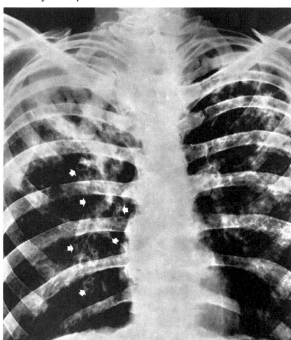

the bloodstream, and throughout the body. Within 3 to 6 weeks, the body's immune system usually controls the infection and arrests the disease. But if the infection reactivates, it can spread rapidly throughout the lungs, destroying lung tissue and causing serious respiratory problems, and can eventually invade other organs as well.

Signs and symptoms
TB usually produces no symptoms at first, or may cause fever, fatigue, malaise, and weight loss so gradual as to go unnoticed. It's typically discovered through a chest X-ray, which shows tubercles and lung tissue damage. Eventually, or with reactivation, more pronounced symptoms develop: coughing, at first dry but later with increased amounts of thick mucus and possibly blood, chest pains, pronounced fatigue, headaches, and increased difficulty in breathing. However, the course of TB

varies widely; some persons with extensive lung damage may show no symptoms, and some highly infectious persons may remain in relatively good health for many years.

Treatment and prevention
Fortunately, drug treatment usually cures TB, although treatment must be continued for 9 to 18 months or longer. But after 2 to 4 weeks of treatment, the disease is no longer contagious, and an infected person can resume normal activities while continuing drug therapy.

Persons at high risk for TB and those who cannot avoid exposure to TB, such as overseas military personnel and Peace Corps volunteers, may benefit from immunization with bacille Calmette-Guérin (BCG) vaccine. BCG provides active immunity against TB; although it doesn't prevent infection, it greatly reduces an infection's effects.

A deadly and unexpected disease

The mysterious Legionnaires' disease, which appeared suddenly in July 1976 at an American Legion convention in Philadelphia, is actually a kind of bacterial pneumonia. Fortunately, the microbe responsible has been identified, and effective antibiotics are available. We now know this microbe thrives in cool, quiet water; consequently, new standards have been established for the design and regular cleaning of air conditioning and humidifying equipment.

who try succeeds in completely giving up the habit. But if you smoke, quitting is the single most effective step you can take toward better health and longer life. So quitting is worth all the will and imagination you can put into it.

Here are some ways to quit smoking:

Cutting down. Gradually reducing the amount you smoke each day works for some people. After all, this is the way you started smoking only run in reverse. Many smokers find, however, that reduction never seems to arrive at zero cigarettes each day; a gradual rebuilding of the habit to former levels often happens instead.

Quitting cold. This is the method for heroes. If you can get through 3 or 4 days of sudden cigarette withdrawal, you can probably get through the rest of your life without cigarettes. You may have symptoms of sudden withdrawal, though: anxiety, insomnia, irritability, intestinal problems, and others. Quitting cold requires some self-preparation, too. Pick a day, muster your willpower, and try to imagine your daily routine as it will be without smoking. You should allow for several weeks before quitting to work on changing your smoker's image of yourself into a nonsmoker's image.

Drugs and nicotine substitutes. No tranquilizer, narcotic antagonist (which nullifies the effects of a habit-forming drug), or safe nicotine substitute has proven any more effective in stopping the smoking

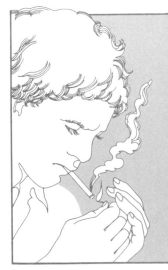

The frightening chemical complexity of smoke

If you're a smoker, perhaps you've never thought much about the chemical makeup of smoke. About 1,000 different chemical compounds have been identified in cigarette smoke, everything from fatty acids and alcohols to poisonous gases such as carbon monoxide, cyanide, and oxides of nitrogen. A burning cigarette resembles nothing so much as a miniature chemical factory, turning out nicotine at an immense cost in toxic wastes.

habit than a placebo (an inactive substance, such as sugar, disguised to resemble a real drug). Of course, even placebos have helped some people quit smoking—as long as you believe something works, it generally does.

*Aversion therapy.*Associating unpleasant experiences (often electric shocks) with smoking is a logical but somewhat traumatic way to break the habit. Ask your doctor about this technique and for information concerning various aversion programs. You may think, with justification, that this technique sounds like a last resort. Given the importance to you of giving up smoking, you shouldn't dismiss anything that works.

*Hypnosis.*Consult your doctor for an opinion and a recommendation to a reliable hypnotist. Hypnotic suggestion certainly has helped many people to quit, but susceptibility to hypnosis varies greatly among different subjects. Hypnosis may not be right for you.

*Gadgets and gimmicks.*To ease the yearning you may feel at first for a cigarette, divert yourself with anything that keeps your attention focused elsewhere: try crossword puzzles, knitting, brisk walks, going to movies, shopping, swimming, running, cycling; take up a wind instrument or any activity to keep your hands, mind, and body busy. Put fake cigarettes, toothpicks, or cinnamon sticks in your mouth, if that helps (but try not to increase your food intake). True, you may acquire a toothpick habit, but it's cheaper and safer than cigarettes.

Index